Alternative Therapy Sequel: 11

Essentials of Trace Elements & Biochemic Medicine

By

Prof. Dr. Debasish Kundu

M.D.H., F.F.Hom, F.I.H.M.S., Ph.D.(U.S.A.), D.Sc.(Colombo)

Edited By

Prof. Seyed Farzin Hassanzadeh Salehian

M.D., Diploma TCM, Ph.D., D.Sc.

Originals

Delhi

First Edition 2017

ISBN 13: 978-81-8454-186-1

ISBN 10: 81-8454-186-4

Published By

Originals

A-6, Second Floor, Nimri Commercial Centre,
Ashok Vihar Phase-4, Delhi - 110 052 (India)
Tel.: +91 11 2730 2453 Fax: 011 4706 1936
Website: www.Lppindia.com
e-mail: info@Lppindia.com

Printed At

D K Fine Art Press P Ltd.
Delhi-110052

Printed in India

Prof. Dr. Debasish Kundu

M.D.H., F.F.Hom, F.I.H.M.S., Ph.D.(U.S.A.), D.Sc.(Colombo)

Fellow of International Holistic Medical Society, CA, U.S.A.

Fellow of Foundation of Homeopathy, MO, U.S.A.

Fellow of World E.Homeopathy System of Medical Council, Hong Kong

Faculty, International Holistic Medical Society, CA, U.S.A.

Vice-President, American Nutritional Medical Association, CA, U.S.A.

Visiting Professor, Khulna Homeopathic Medical College & Hospital, Khulna, Bangladesh

World Vice President, International Elite University, Cagliari, Italy & California, USA.

Recipient, Royal Assyrian Order of Merit

Laureate, Dag Hammarskjold Award for Medicine

Editor In Chief, International Journal of Homeopathy & Natural Medicines, USA

Editor in Chief, The Internet Journal of Herbal and Plant Medicine, U.S.A.

Author,

Materia Medica for the New Age Man,

Diseases of Women,

Natural Medicines,

A Clinical Treatise on Cancer,

Aids & Homeopathy,

Pharmacodynamics in Spagyric Medicine (Plant Alchemy),

Aids & Your Sex Life,

Aids & Homeopathy,

Essentials of Acupuncture, etc.

Prof. Seyed Farzin Hassanzadeh Salehian M.D.

Diploma TCM, Ph.D., D.Sc.

Unesco Representative for Iran,

Faculty, Harvard University and Oxford University,

President, International Elite University, Cagliari, Italy & California, USA

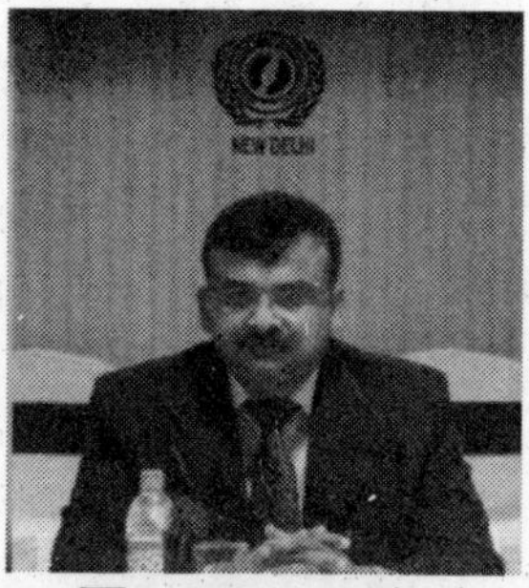

Foreword

I am pleased to have the opportunity to write foreword for the book of Essentials of Trace Elements & Bioplasgens (Incl. Relationship with Spagyrics) which is written by Dr. Debasish Kundu for ADEH students. Because I have a dream for all my Electro Homoeopathic practitioners that one day they must get an official Certificate from any Government Agency and I am happy to say that Maharashtra is the First State in India to offer an Official Electro Homoeopathy Certificate which is being awarded by the Government Agency. Also I have some friends who helped me to fulfill my dream to introduce a Government recognised ADVANCE DIPLOMA IN ELECTRO HOMOEOPATHY (ADEH) course in Maharashtra.

When word comes "ADVANCED" means something new and scientific, so while reading the contents of the book, I found something new and advanced. Since long time Dr. Kundu is writing books on different subjects which are very easy to understand and rich in contents, so I believe this book will help all the Students, Practitioners & Lovers of Electro-Homoeopathy besides students in perusing ADEH examination which contains the study material mentioned in Syllabus by MSBVE, Mumbai. This entire course material will help to improve the knowledge in Electro Homoeopathy subject.

Dr. Trideep Guha
BPTH, MD (ECH) MBA, Ph.D., MRCE (USA)
Chairman
Educational & Medical/Paramedical Council of India
Executive Member:
Paramedical Syllabus Committee,
MSBVEE, Mumbai (Govt. of Maharashtra)

Email id
drtrideep.g@gmail.com, empci@hotmail.com
Visit us at :
www.empci.com

Published By

Originals

A-6, Second Floor, Nimri Commercial Centre,
Ashok Vihar Phase-4, Delhi - 110 052 (India)
Tel.: +91 11 2730 2453 Fax: 011 4706 1936
Website: www.Lppindia.com
e-mail: info@Lppindia.com

In Association with

ADEH PRACTISIONERS ASSOCIATION MAHARASHTRA

N-123, Second floor, Infront of Devanjali flats,
Reshimbag, City & District : Nagpur
State : Maharashtra Country : INDIA
Phone : +91-712-2700606, +91-712-2700651, +91-712-2700777

Contents

Preface

Cell Salts or Bioplasgens have always been considered an important part of healing in Homeopathy and Spagyrics. The methods of preparation of Biochemic and Homeopathic Trituration remedies are quite identical.

According to Dr. Schuessler, the Father of Biochemic Medicine, a deficiency of a certain cell salt gives rise to certain symptoms which point to its use as a remedy, and cure is affected by the restoration of the equilibrium of the salt in the body. The modern biological findings tell us of Chelation or salt-hunger as one of the potential disease causing factor. According to Dr. Schuessler Homeopathy works indirectly through Biochemic principles, since many Homeopathic remedies contain one or more of the cell salts. The greater the proportion of a salt in a (homeopathic) remedy, the greater the resemblance between the two (e.g. Pulsatilla and Kali Sulph, which both have among their leading indications, aggravation in a warm room and in the evenings, and amelioration in the open air.) Both Aconite and Arnica contain Ferrum Phos and the similarities between the remedies are to be considered. Likewise there are many common features between Hepar Sulph and Calc Sulph. Schuessler opined that Biochemistry rectifies disease directly, by the administration of homogeneous substances.

According to Schuessler human body is composed of two kinds of materials ; organic and inorganic. The former is more essential to life than the latter. The chemical compounds of living things are known as organic compounds. Friedrich

Wöhler a German chemist who lived in the 1800s is considered the father of organic chemistry. All organic compounds contain carbon. Carbon is so important to the structure of organic molecules that organic chemistry has been called the study of carbon and its compounds. Other elements are readily incorporated into organic molecules, though the determining feature of an organic molecule is the presence or absence of carbon atoms.

Organic molecules are sometimes able to incorporate other elements as integral parts of their working structure. An example of this is in hemoglobin, which is a type of organic molecule called a protein. Specifically, haemoglobin is a metalloprotein, which means it incorporates atoms of iron into its active site to better capture and transport oxygen in red blood cells.

Inorganic compounds are those that lack long carbon chains at their core. While some inorganic compounds contain carbon, they do not contain carbon that is bonded to hydrogen. Inorganic compounds include substances such as salt, carbon dioxide and water. Inorganic compounds are important chemicals for many organisms. For example, all living organisms require copious amounts of water and salt in small quantities.

The inorganic constituents are water and certain cell salts. The relative quantities in the human organism are as follows: water 7/10th, cell salts 1/20th and the remainder is the organic matters. Though so small, these cell salts are a confirmed vital portion of our body structure. Water and organic matter are used by these salts in building up the cells of the body.

This book contains all essential materials concerning Trace Elements & Bioplasgen and their Clinical Materia Medica with useful suggestions.

Dr. Debasish Kundu
drdkundu@msn.com

Part I

1

Introduction to Trace Elements & Bioplasgens

It all began way back towards the end of the nineteenth century when a German physician, Dr. Wilhelm Heinrich Schuessler wrote on article on his theory of biochemistry.

The human body, according to him, was made up of these twelve inorganic substances or cell salts. Each of which had very specific functions in the body. They exist – in a perfect state – in perfect balance within each body, combining with organic substances in order to maintain the body's cells and keep all the many body functions going. If there was any deficiency in any cell salt, it upset this delicate and wonderful balance and the result was ill health. What lead him to this conclusion that there were twelve salts that were most important? This was because when a body was burned, what was left, when analysed were these cell salts.

Schuessler saw the inorganic salts as the body's builders and the organic substances as the building blocks. For perfect health, there had to be perfect teamwork of all the twelve builders and if any one fell behind, it had to be given a boost and brought back to its original state. The essence of a healthy life is to balance, regulate and restore the cells of the body naturally to promote self healing. Mineral Tissue Salts or Bioplasgens are the 'Vital, essential mineral' building blocks of the body. They promote and enhance optimum assimilation and utilization of nutrients consumed in our daily diet.

The word 'Biochemistry' comes from the Greek 'Bios' for 'Life', coupled with 'Chemistry', the science that studies the composition of elements and the changes they go through. In the therapeutic sphere, Biochemistry is the system of treatment that uses the tissue remedies (inorganic salts of the body tissues) as medicine.

The biochemical therapy uses the Tissue Salts to normalise cell health, redress an imbalance and stimulate the immune system response of the body. The health of the human body depends upon the health of each of its cell, its metabolic processes within the cells.

When one or more of these elements become deficient the normal cell function or metabolism is disturbed. This is known as disease.

When certain mineral constituents or Tissue Salts are deficient, the ability of the cells to assimilate, to excrete and use nutrition becomes upset. Cell nutrition and cell metabolism could be returned to normalcy by supplying the right Tissue Salt in a low potency (usually 3x).

According to biochemistry, roughly 96 percent of the mass of the human body is made up of just four elements: oxygen, carbon, hydrogen and nitrogen, with a lot of that in the form of water. The remaining 4 percent is a sparse sampling of the periodic table of elements.

Some of the more prominent representatives are called macro nutrients, whereas those appearing only at the level of parts per million or less are referred to as micronutrients.

These nutrients perform various functions, including the building of bones and cell structures, regulating the body's pH, carrying charge, and driving chemical reactions.

Here's a look at the chemical composition of the human body, including element abundance and how each element is used. Elements are listed in order of decreasing abundance, with the most common element (by mass) listed first. Approximately 96% of body weight consists of only four elements: oxygen, carbon, hydrogen, and nitrogen. Calcium, phosphorus, magnesium, sodium, potassium, chlorine, and sulfur are macronutrients or elements the body needs in a significant amount.

1. Oxygen

Liquid oxygen is blue. By mass, oxygen is the most abundant element in the human body. If you think about it, this makes sense, since most of the body consists of water or H2O. Oxygen accounts for 61-65% of the mass of the human body. Even though there are many more atoms of hydrogen in your body than oxygen, each oxygen atom is 16 times more massive than a hydrogen atom.

2. Carbon

All living organisms contain carbon, which forms the basis for all of the organic molecules in the body. Carbon is the second most abundant element in the human body, accounting for 18% of body weight.

All organic molecules (fats, proteins, carbohydrates, nucleic acids) contain carbon. Carbon also is found as carbon dioxide or CO2. You inhale air that contains about 20% oxygen. Air you exhale contains much less oxygen, but is rich in carbon dioxide.

3. Hydrogen

Hydrogen accounts for 10% of the mass of the human body.

Since around 60% of your body weight is water, much of the hydrogen exists in water, which functions to transport nutrients, remove wastes, lubricate organs and joints, and regulate body temperature. Hydrogen is also important in energy production and use. The H+ ion can be used as a hydrogen ion or proton pump to produce ATP and regulate numerous chemical reactions. All organic molecules contain hydrogen in addition to carbon.

4. Nitrogen

Approximately 3% of the mass of the human body is nitrogen.

Proteins, nucleic acids, and other organic molecules contain nitrogen. Nitrogen gas is found in the lungs, since the primary gas in air is nitrogen.

5. Calcium

Calcium accounts for 1.5% of human body weight. Calcium is a metal. It readily oxidizes in air. Because it makes up such a large part of the skeleton, about one-third of the mass of human body comes from calcium, after water has been removed.

Calcium is used to give the skeletal system its rigidity and strength. Calcium is found in bones and teeth. The Ca^{2+} ion is important for muscle function.

6. Phosphorus

About 1.2% to 1.5% of your body consists of phosphorus. White phosphorus powder glows green in the presence of oxygen. Although the term "phosphorescence" refers to phosphorus, the glow of white phosphorus as it oxidizes is really a form of chemiluminescence.

Phosphorus is important for bone structure and is part of the primary energy molecule in the body, ATP or adenosine triphosphate. Most of the phosphorus in the body is in the bones and teeth.

7. Potassium

Potassium makes up 0.2% to 0.35% of the adult human body.

Potassium is a soft, silvery-white metal that quickly oxidizes. Potassium is an important mineral in all cells. It functions as an electrolyte and is particularly important for conducting electrical impulses and for muscle contraction.

8. Sulfur

Sulfur's abundance is 0.20% to 0.25% in the human body. Pure sulfur is a yellow nonmetallic element.

Sulfur is an important component of amino acids and proteins. It's present in keratin, which forms skin, hair, and nails. It's also needed for cellular respiration, allowing cells to use oxygen.

9. Sodium

Approximately 0.10% to 0.15% of your body mass is the element sodium.

Sodium is an important electrolyte in the body. It is an important component of cellular fluids and is needed for the transmission of nerve impulses. It helps regulate fluid volume, temperature, and blood pressure.

10. Magnesium

The metal magnesium comprises about 0.05% of human body weight.

However, this does not exhaust the list of elements that you need. Sulfur is not usually mentioned as a dietary supplement because the body gets plenty of it in proteins.

And there are several other elements — such as silicon, boron, nickel, vanadium and lead — that may play a biological role and their deficiencies lead to serious diseases, diabetes when chromium and vanadium are deficient.

"*This may be due to the fact that a biochemical function has not been defined by experimental evidence*," said Victoria Drake from the Linus Pauling Institute at Oregon State University.

A normal diet consists of thousands of compounds (some containing trace elements) whose effects are the study of ongoing research. For now, we can only say for certain what 20 or so elements are doing. Here is a quick rundown, with the percentage of body weight in parentheses.

Oxygen (65%) and hydrogen (10%) are predominantly found in water, which makes up about 60 percent of the body by weight. It's practically impossible to imagine life without water.

Carbon (18%) is synonymous with life. Its central role is due to the fact that it has four bonding sites that allow for the building of long, complex chains of molecules. Moreover, carbon bonds can be formed and broken with a modest amount of energy, allowing for the dynamic organic chemistry that goes on in our cells.

Nitrogen (3%) is found in many organic molecules, including the amino acids that make up proteins, and the nucleic acids that make up DNA.

Calcium (1.5%) is the most common mineral in the human body — nearly all of it found in bones and teeth. Ironically, calcium's most important role is in bodily functions, such as muscle contraction and protein regulation. In fact, the body will actually pull calcium from bones (causing problems like osteoporosis) if there's not enough of the element in a person's diet.

Phosphorus (1%) is found predominantly in bone but also in the molecule ATP, which provides energy in cells for driving chemical reactions.

Potassium (0.25%) is an important electrolyte (meaning it carries a charge in solution). It helps regulate the heartbeat and is vital for electrical signaling in nerves.

Sulfur (0.25%) is found in two amino acids that are important for giving proteins their shape.

Sodium (0.15%) is another electrolyte that is vital for electrical signaling in nerves. It also regulates the amount of water in the body.

Chlorine (0.15%) is usually found in the body as a negative ion, called chloride. This electrolyte is important for maintaining a normal balance of fluids.

Magnesium (0.05%) plays an important role in the structure of the skeleton and muscles. It also is necessary in more than 300 essential metabolic reactions.

Iron (0.006%) is a key element in the metabolism of almost all living organisms. It is also found in hemoglobin, which is the oxygen carrier in red blood cells. Half of women don't get enough iron in their diet.

Fluorine (0.0037%) is found in teeth and bones. Outside of preventing tooth decay, it does not appear to have any importance to bodily health.

Zinc (0.0032%) is an essential trace element for all forms of life. Several proteins contain structures called "zinc fingers" help to regulate genes. Zinc deficiency has been known to lead to dwarfism in developing countries.

Copper (0.0001%) is important as an electron donor in various biological reactions. Without enough copper, iron won't work properly in the body.

Iodine (0.000016%) is required for making of thyroid hormones, which regulate metabolic rate and other cellular functions. Iodine deficiency, which can lead to goiter and brain damage, is an important health problem throughout much of the world.

Selenium (0.000019%) is essential for certain enzymes, including several anti-oxidants. Unlike animals, plants do not appear to require selenium for survival, but they do absorb it, so there are several cases of selenium poisoning from eating plants grown in selenium-rich soils.

Chromium (0.0000024%) helps regulate sugar levels by interacting with insulin, but the exact mechanism is still not completely understood.

Manganese (0.000017%) is essential for certain enzymes, in particular those that protect mitochondria — the place where usable energy is generated inside cells — from dangerous oxidants.

Molybdenum (0.000013%) is essential to virtually all life forms. In humans, it is important for transforming sulfur into a usable form. In nitrogen-fixing bacteria, it is important for transforming nitrogen into a usable form.

Cobalt (0.0000021%) is contained in vitamin B12, which is important in protein formation and DNA regulation. The cell is the basic structural and functional unit of all known living organisms. It is the smallest unit of life that is classified as a living thing, and is often called the building block of life.

An average human body (weighing 70 kg), contains a small amount of pure gold. The average person's body weighing 70 kilograms would contain a total mass of 0.2 milligrams of gold. Gold plays a vital role in both the health and maintenance of the joints, as well as being a key element in the transmittal of electrical signals throughout the body, also, it had to do with making the electrical connections that allow the heart to beat. Of interesting note, the human body contains 1.0 gram of Silicon. This element is commonly found in the presence of gold in nature and its metabolic function is currently unknown.

Organisms can be classified as unicellular (consisting of a single cell; including most bacteria) or multicellular (including plants and animals). Humans contain about 10 trillion (10) cells. Most plant and animal cells are between 1 and 100 µm and therefore are visible only under the microscope. The cell was discovered by Robert Hooke in 1665.

The cell theory, first developed in 1839 by Matthias Jakob Schleiden and Theodor Schwann, states that all organisms are composed of one or more cells, that all cells come from preexisting cells, that vital functions of an organism occur within cells, and that all cells contain the hereditary information necessary for regulating cell functions and for transmitting information to the next generation of cells.

Cells are the building blocks of the body. All our internal organs our skin our blood all made up of cells. The health of our body is dependent upon the health of the smallest part of our body; the cell.

Our cells are replaced cyclically on a regular basis. When the cell does not have the proper materials that it needs to be a healthy cell, our overall health suffers. Cell Salts provide the components that our cells need to be healthy. Taken on a regular basis over a period of time our cells rebuild themselves with the proper healthy materials that we need.

It was also found as well that the cell salts provide remedies for many illnesses, not as a medicine, but as an enhancer for the health of the body on a cell level, helping the body to heal itself.

Cell salts are nutritional preparations of certain mineral compounds found within all living things. Twelve in number, cell salts are an extremely versatile, natural healing method.

In 1873, German biochemist, William H. Schuessler found that there are certain essential minerals that the body requires. He discovered this by studying the remains of numerous cadavers and examining them after calcinations or burning to see what essential elements remained.

He found that an imbalance or a lack of any of these minerals may lead to disease in the tissues so lacking. Providing the missing minerals to the tissues corrects that imbalance and so eliminates the illness.

Thus the cell salts provide a rebalancing of the body enabling its natural disease controlling mechanisms to function. To this end, the cell salts are not a "cure" or a medicine *per se* but a body function balancing supplement albeit a powerful one nonetheless.

Schuessler found that according to the time of year we are born we are deficient in three of the cell salts. Replenishing that deficiency through micro cell nutrients greatly improves the health of the body.

'that branch of science which treats of the composition of animal and vegetable matter, the process by which the various fluids and tissues are formed; the nature and cause of the abnormal condition called disease and restoration to health by supplying to the body the deficient cell salts.'

—Dr. W.Schuessler

It has been found that the cell salts provide remedies for many illnesses, not as a medicine, but as an enhancer for the health of the body on a cell level, helping the body to heal itself.

Cell salts are nutritional preparations of certain mineral compounds found within all living things. Twelve in number, cell salts are an extremely versatile, natural healing method.

This system of Medicine is based upon the "cell theory" of Virchow in 1858. He said that the body is a collection of cells and that all medical treatment should center around the health of the individual cell. This system of medicine is based on cellular health.

The importance of the inorganic components of cells were recognized, hence the 12 salts were found to be the basic building blocks of the cell and water and other organic substances were used by the salts in building the cells of the body.

If there is a deficiency in any of these salts the cell and consequently the body would suffer.

These 12 salts are essential for the health and growth of the body. They are grouped in fours; Phosphates, Chlorides, Sulphates, and Fluorides (also Silica).

The 12 salts are as follows; Calcium Phosphate, Ferrum Phosphate, Kali Phosphate, Natrum Phosphate, Kali Mr., Natrum Mur, Calcium Sulph, Natrum Sulph, Kali Sulph, Calcium Fluor, and Silica.

These 12 salts were found to make up the human body.

Due to the minute scale of cells, the ideal way to replenish any deficiency is through very small micronutrients that go directly to the depleted cells.

Tinctures of the salts provide an easily absorbed transport for the body, enabling the needed salts to go directly to the bloodstream without the body expending much needed energy in digesting and processing the micronutrient cell salts.

More people are finding out the benefits of the salts and the 12 remedies.

The Salts now sold commercially are in lactose pill form, and the minerals salts are manufactured in a lab.

However, there are a lot of lactose intolerant people and those persons cannot use the lactose pills without consequences.

There is another alternative, that of the tincture or liquid form of the salts dissolved into an alcohol base, much like a lot of herbal tinctures are. These salts are dissolved into grain alcohol in the same triturations as the pill form.

The advantage of taking a tincture as opposed to the pill is that it allows for an even more rapid absorption into the bloodstream.

2

The Functions of The Cell

Cells are composed of three basic parts, a nucleus, or brain of the cell, the cytoplasm, which provides nourishment to the cell's nucleus, and the cell membrane, which contains both and gives it form and protection. At about two months of age, your body has all the cells it will ever get, somewhere around one hundred trillion of them.

For the rest of your life, your body will not produce any additional cells, only replace the old cells.

Also, your cells are constantly in the process of dying and being replaced, at the rate of three hundred million per minute.

So every four weeks, your entire outer layer of skin is replaced. Every two months, practically every cell in your heart muscle is rebuilt.

Within two to three years, your entire bone structure is replaced. So every two to three years, every cell in your body is replaced with a new cell.

In other words, you'll have a totally new body.

The question is, what kind of body will it be? Will your new body be weaker or stronger than the one you have today?

It's up to you. Because as your old cells die and are replaced, your new cells depend totally upon the building materials you provide it – the foods you eat, the liquids you drink and the air you breathe.

If your cell's needs are properly met, then ultimately a new, healthy and strong cell will be reproduced.

So if you want energy, physical strength and freedom from disease, then take care of your cells.

The cell is a chemical factory in which hundreds of chemical reactions take place. The "brain" or nucleus of the cell controls everything that goes on in this factory.

It is a necessary function of the cell membrane to let in proper nutrients to fuel this factory and keep out all harmful substances like bacteria and viruses.

Energy is produced through the burning of oxygen and sugar in the cell. The catalyst for this process is in the form of an enzyme. The enzyme gathers necessary raw material for the reactions to take place and acts as a catalyst for the reaction. Should that enzyme be lacking the exact sequence of reactions is not possible and the cell cannot survive.

The enzymes in a cell wear out after a while. The nucleus acts as a template to produce more enzymes. The enzymes must be constructed out of basic materials, namely proteins, vitamins, and minerals. If your diet is deficient in these ingredients then the cell cannot properly replenish the enzymes. The chemical factory comes to a halt and the cell dies.

Hence, you must get all the trace elements needed on a daily basis.

Energy and information are two terms used to describe the same thing. Even the simplest processes in our body need salt, or its inherent elements (ionized energy). Our nervous system is really a sophisticated energy network. It transmits stimulation that is recorded via sensory input (all of our senses are actually energy receptors, our eyes receive waves of energy, information in the form of light frequencies, our ears receive sound frequencies or patterns of energy and our nose senses odors, also electrical charges in the atmosphere) Everything in the universe works by the fundamental principles of energy! Anyway, these sensory inputs that travel to our brain are passed on to our muscles in order for them to react to the respective stimuli (electrical current).

An electric potential occurs on the membrane wall of a cell when the positively charged potassium ions leave the cells and the positively charged sodium ions cannot enter due to their size. The outside becomes positively charged and the inside, negatively charged. When a nerve cell is stimulated, its membrane suddenly becomes polar opposite and is permeable for the sodium ions, allowing the electrical charge to enter. Without the elements of potassium and sodium in salt, none of this is possible. Not even a single thought, let alone an action, is possible without their presence. First comes the thought, a wave of energy received in the brain. This thought is nothing more than an electromagnetic frequency. The salt is responsible for enabling this frequency to transmit commands to the muscles and organs.

The cytoplasm contains all the basic bioplasgens. Different types of cells require more or less of certain of the salts, for example nerve cells require larger amounts of Kali Phosphate to function and blood cells higher amounts of Ferrum phosphate.

Although proper nutrition of course is also important to the health of the body and cells, vitamin supplements and diet often overlook these essential micro nutrients salts that the cells need to remain healthy.

Now Many of the bodies processes are electrically charged processes. Cell enzymes work to attract the necessary raw materials by electrical attraction.

It is well documented that the electromagnetic energy of the Moon have an effect upon the earth and tides. We, as residents of the Earth, cannot help but be influenced by the electromagnetism of our external environment. So too, the cellular factory of our bodies. The enzymes attracting the materials it needs by electrical attraction.

Therefore all living things are affected by the cosmic influences surrounding us.

At the moment of our birth we are affected by the electromagnetic rays bombarding us and the Earth sphere. And evidence suggests that our very brain patterns are affected by the planets surrounding us at the moment of birth, dictating our personality and tendencies. It is not difficult to assume that our basic physical functions are also affected by these electromagnetic influences.

In fact, Schuessler found in his studies that according to the month that we are born, we have a deficiency of at least 3 of the salts due to being in the womb for 9 months, we are deficient in the remaining months making up the 12 months.

Dr. George W. Carey, related them to the 12 signs of the zodiac, noting that the sign on the Eastern horizon, or your rising sign greatly influenced the balance of these essential salts in the cells.

3

Astrology and Bioplasgens

It is a scientifically established fact that we are constantly bombarded by electromagnetic rays from the Moon, the Sun and the stars. These rays are affecting every living thing on the planet, including ocean tides, weather and the growth cycles of the Earth. Astrology is based on the concept that we are the centre of our own personal Universe – that we are the Sun, so to speak – and that the horizon at the time and place of our birth revolves around us. This places a unique stamp upon us at birth, determining our personality and tendencies upon arrival into physical existence, i.e. the electromagnetic energies stamp a pattern into the energy configurations of our brain. Studies have been undertaken in Japan which examine the effects of the time of year upon chemical processes and reactions. It was found that the conditions of the Earth's electromagnetic fields influenced the rate of reaction. This also confirms the ancient alchemists' insistence that the time of year would influence the outcome of an operation. In the perspective of astrology each of the twelve signs of the zodiac ; viz., Aries, Taurus, Gemini, Cancer, Leo, Virgo, Libra, Scorpio, Sagittarius, Capricorn, Aquarius, and Pisces – corresponds to a time of the year, beginning with Aries at the spring equinox and ending with Pisces. The individual astrological chart alters the original pattern according to the horizon surrounding the individual at the time of birth, so that not every sign is in its proper house, i.e. Aries first, Pisces twelfth.

Astrology has long since discarded as pseudoscience. But new scientific research suggests our zodiac sign actually may have more to do with our health than one might think. This is not because of the influence of any heavenly bodies, but because of the time of the year one is born. A new study suggests that our birth month has a connection with the diseases we might develop in our lifetime.

Mary Regina Boland, Nicholas Tatonetti and other researchers at the Columbia University Department of Medicine examined records for an incredible 1.75 million patients born between 1900 and 2000 who had been treated at Columbia University Medical Center. Using statistical analysis, they combed through 1,688 different diseases and found 55 that had a correlation with birth month, including ADHD, reproductive performance, asthma, eyesight and ear infections.

The researchers emphasize that other environmental factors, such as diet, medical care and exercise, are more likely to influence whether one acquires a disease.

The researchers found that being born in June, August, January and December provided no big advantage or disadvantage when it came to disease. Other months, such as October and November, were associated with increased risk of disease, while the months of February, March, April, May and July tended to be associated with decreased disease risk.

People who are born in December are quite possibly healthier than the rest of us-and a lot healthier than those born in March.

Those with December birthdays are predisposed to respiratory syncytial virus, and infection that causes pneumonia, but that's nothing compared to people who are born in March, who are predisposed to a veritable medical textbook of illnesses and disorders: Alzheimer's, schizophrenia, autism, narcolepsy, Hodgkin's disease, multiple sclerosis, bipolar disorder, and epilepsy.

Medical experts from a variety of prestigious research institutions, including Stanford University, Southwest Missouri State University, and Stanley Medical Research Institute in Bethesda, MD., have independently found a link between the month in which you were born and predisposition to certain illnesses, reports ABC News. If there is any explanation between birth month and disease it is most likely environmental, although no study has been able to prove a definitive cause-and-effect relationship. For example, fetal exposure to a virus in the second trimester of pregnancy when neuro-development begins may be linked to schizophrenia.

It is summarized below:

January

Alzheimer's, schizophrenia, respiratory syncytal virus, heart problems, hypertension, or high blood pressure.

February

Alzheimer's, schizophrenia, bipolar disorder, epilepsy.

March

Alzheimer's, schizophrenia, autism, narcolepsy, Hodgkin's disease, multiple sclerosis, bipolar disorder, epilepsy, Prostate cancer, atrial fibrillation, congestive cardiac failure.

April

Leukemia, dyslexia, learning disabilities, multiple sclerosis, Parkinson's disease, bipolar disorder, epilepsy, Angina, ALS.

May

Dyslexia, learning disabilities, multiple sclerosis, ALS, Parkinson's disease.

June

Anorexia, diabetes, dyslexia, learning disabilities, multiple sclerosis, ALS, Heart diseases, Parkinson's disease, and celiac disease.

July

Diabetes, celiac disease, dyslexia, learning disabilities.

August

Diabetes, celiac disease, autism, Crohn's disease.

September

ADHD, asthma, Allergy-related diseases.

October

Asthma, eczema, Overall health issues.

November

Asthma, eczema, respiratory syncytial virus, ADHD and respiratory diseases.

December

Respiratory syncytial virus, bumps and bruising.

The medical experts opine that while there appears to be a pattern between birth month and disease, none of this is a prediction for what will happen to specific individuals. In addition, more research is needed to figure out how a person's birth month actually influences his or her health.

Hippocrates, the father of modern medicine, wrote that "*A physician cannot safely administer medicine if he is unacquainted with astrology*" (Chapter 3, page 81; *Astrology and Your Health* by Jeanne Avery, Published by Paraview, 2004) So a physician shouldn't do anything without checking in with the Earth cycles first or the treatment could fail or have complications.

That is an analogy as to how Astrology works. Not your average horoscope in the daily newspaper, it is much more than that. Used properly it is the Operators Manual to ourselves to guide us to our purpose in this life and to show us our predispositions to ailments and imbalances in our bodies as well as other levels.

It is divided into twelve slices of a pie so to speak. The twelve signs of the zodiac, Aries, Taurus, Gemini, Cancer, Leo, Virgo, Libra, Scorpio, Sagittarius, Capricorn, Aquarius, Pisces. Each corresponds to months of the year starting with spring equinox, Aries and ending with Pisces.

The Individual Chart alters the original pattern according to the horizon around the person at the time of birth so that not every sign is in its "proper" house. Aries being 1st, Pisces the 12th. This interplay of energies is what makes each one unique. The House is the playing field, or the "where" the energies are operating. The Planet in the house is "What" is operating, and the Sign on the cusp of the house is the "How" of it. These can be benefic, or easy and compatible, or malefic, which is a struggle. "Bad" aspects are challenges we present to ourselves to work out here.

Anyway, this is not the place to go into an in depth lesson in Astrology. Suffice to say it all involves subtle and physical energies that affect each person uniquely.

Basically the Sun's position in a chart, influences body chemistry. Saturn is also important to Health.

The South Node of the Moon, calculated by the time of day of birth is also important as to which bioplasgen regimen he/she falls. It is summarised below:

Zodiac Sign	**Bioplasgen**
Aquarius (21 January- 19 February)	Natrum Muriaticum
Cancer (22 June-23 July)	Calcarea Flourica

Capricorn (22 December-20 January)	Calcarea Phosphorica
Scorpio (24 October-22 November)	Calcarea Sulphurica
Pisces (20 February-20 March)	Ferrum Phosphoricum
Gemini (22 May-21 June)	Kalium Muriaticum
Aries (21 March-20 April)	Kalium Phosphoricum
Virgo (24 August-23 September)	Kalium Sulphuricum
Leo (24 July-23 August)	Magnesia Phosphorica
Libra (24 September-23 October)	Natrum Phosphoricum
Taurus (21 April-21 May)	Natrum Sulphuricum
Sagittarius (20 November-21 December)	Silicea

The cell salts that you will need to take will be the ones that correspond to each of the above components of your zodiac. There are three for each sun sign, these are your 'bridge salts'.

Schuessler observed that depending on the time of year you are born, you are deficient in at least three of the salts that he theorized would have been made up if we spent the whole 12 months in the womb. Hence the three 'bridge' salts for your sun sign.

In addition to the salts being an excellent way to supplement and balance the body according to your own tendencies, they are also an excellent and safe way to treat minor ailments of the body.

The cell salts may be used by themselves for the remedies listed or to benefit certain organ systems and functions of the body. They may also be used in combination with each other to treat specific symptoms.

Cell Salts can be combined to effect a more complete healing of a condition. They are safe to use on Children and Animals as well.

Placed under the tongue, they are quickly absorbed into the body. Or you can take them in a small amount of water if you prefer.

Generally to heal a condition you may want to take it more frequently than you would as a supplement.

4

Minerals

Mineral salts are responsible for structural functions involving the skeleton and soft tissues and for regulatory functions including neuromuscular transmission, blood clotting, oxygen transport, and enzymatic activity. Calcium, phosphorus, and magnesium are required in relatively large amounts and are designated as macrominerals. These are discussed in this chapter. Minerals needed in smaller amounts are called trace elements; Calcium is the most abundant mineral in the human body, making up 1.5 to 2% of the total body weight. Approximately 1,200 g of calcium are present in the body of an adult human; more than 99% of that amount is found in bones. All living animals possess powerful mechanisms both to conserve calcium and to maintain constant cellular and extracellular concentrations (Arnaud, 1978, 1988; Exton, 1986). These functions are so vital to survival that during severe dietary deficiency or abnormal losses of calcium from the body, they can demineralize bone to prevent even minor degrees of hypocalcemia (i.e., low plasma calcium). Thus, bone acts as a vital physiological tissue providing a readily available source of calcium for maintenance of normal plasma calcium levels, 50% of which is ionized and physiologically active (Arnaud, 1988).

People need more calcium in their diets when they are forming bone, when intestinal absorption of calcium is impaired, and when there are inordinate losses of calcium to the environment (e.g., through increased renal excretion or lactation). If there is insufficient dietary calcium during bone formation, linear growth will be impeded and peak bone mass may not be achieved. If it is insufficient when intestinal absorption is impaired or when there are inordinate losses, the serum concentration of calcium ion (Ca_2+) can be maintained at normal levels only at the expense of bone calcium (Arnaud, 1988).

Phosphorus, along with calcium, is essential for calcification of bones (85% of body phosphorus is located in the skeleton). The remainder of body phosphorus is needed in soft tissues as a co-factor in myriad enzyme systems essential in the metabolism of carbohydrates, lipids, and proteins. In the form of high-energy phosphate compounds, phosphorus contributes to the metabolic potential. The phosphate ion also plays an important role in acid/base balance.

Of total body magnesium, 60 to 65% is found in bone and 27% is located in muscles (Shils, 1988). Magnesium is second only to potassium as the most predominant cation within cells and is essential both for the functions of many enzyme systems and for neuromuscular transmission.

Minerals that are required in relatively large amounts are called macrominerals to distinguish them from trace elements, minerals needed in smaller amounts. Calcium, phosphorus, and magnesium are macrominerals. Low intakes of calcium, which occur commonly, have been associated with age-related osteoporosis. A dietary deficiency of phosphorus is unlikely, due to its wide distribution in foods. The mean population intake of magnesium, although slightly below the RDA, probably does not represent a health hazard.

Maximum bone mass is achieved by approximately 25 to 30 years of age. It is maintained until 35 to 45 years of age and then declines. Decreased skeletal mass is the most important risk factor for fracture of bones and is a significant public health problem in the United States. One of the problems in assessing the relationship of calcium intake to bone mass is the inherent inaccuracy of dietary recall. In addition, metabolic balance studies, although conducted extensively to determine nutritional requirements for calcium, also have important limitations that prevent accurate determination of the amount of dietary calcium needed to achieve balance.

It is important to achieve peak bone mass because the more mass that is available before age-related loss begins, the less likely it will decrease to a level at which fracture will occur. More dietary calcium is required to achieve peak bone mass than to replace obligatory losses of this ion in urine, feces, and sweat. Thus, people under 25 years of age probably need to ingest sufficient calcium to maintain a positive balance. This quantity will vary from person to person, depending on individual efficiencies of intestinal calcium absorption, but 1,200 mg/day probably provides a margin of safety for almost all normal people ages 11 to 25 years.

Once maximum bone mass is achieved, it is maintained without much change for 10 to 20 years. Calcium intake need not be greater than 800 mg/day during this period, because bone building has been completed and intestinal absorption of calcium is normal. However, men and women lose bone at a constant rate of 0.2 to 0.5% per year, starting at ages 40 to 45. For approximately 10 years immediately before, during, and after menopause, women lose bone more rapidly than men (2 to 5% per year). This rapid rate of bone loss in menopausal women returns to the slower rate shared by the sexes after this 10-year period.

Intestinal calcium absorption and the ability to adapt to low-calcium diets are impaired in many postmenopausal women and elderly people of both sexes. The pathogenesis of these abnormalities is controversial, but evidence suggests that they may be due either to a decreased ability of the kidney to produce the major biologically active metabolite of vitamin D, 1,25 (OH)2D3, such as after menopause, or to absolute decreases in the production of this metabolite due to renal disease, as in old age. The finding that serum levels of immunoreactive and bioactive parathyroid hormone increase with age implies that defects in calcium absorption are functionally important in that they result in sufficient degrees of hypocalcemia to produce chronic secondary hyperparathyroidism—a condition generally associated with bone demineralization. It appears, therefore, that the ability of the intestine to support calcium homeostasis progressively declines with age and that elderly people are increasingly forced to rely on their own bones rather than on the external environment as a source of calcium for maintaining normal extracellular fluid calcium. The degree to which this homeostatic response is needed depends on the severity of the described defects in calcium absorption, the level and bioavailability of dietary calcium, and whether specific therapeutic means are taken to correct defects in calcium absorption.

There is no direct evidence that the impaired intestinal calcium absorption observed during menopause and aging can be overcome by increased calcium intake. Moreover, the evidence that calcium supplementation prevents the trabecular bone loss associated with the menopause is, at best, weak. Thus, calcium supplementation should not be substituted for sex hormone replacement, which prevents postmenopausal bone loss in most women and appears to restore intestinal calcium absorption toward normal. Women taking estrogen replacement should continue to ingest 800 mg of calcium (the RDA). Those menopausal and postmenopausal women at risk for osteoporosis who are unable or refuse to take estrogen may require at least 1,200 mg of calcium per day. Such intakes could delay cortical bone loss and prevent chronic secondary hyperparathyroidism. The association between decreased calcium intake and hypertension is suggestive but inconclusive. The epidemiologic and animal evidence relating calcium to colorectal cancer risk is also inconclusive. High-phosphorus diets may decrease calcium bioavailability, but they also reduce urinary calcium excretion and their influence on bone mass and the risk of osteoporosis is unknown. There are no known adverse effects of magnesium in the amounts currently consumed in the United States, although animal studies show a consistent inverse association between magnesium intake and blood pressure.

5
Trace Elements

Trace elements (or trace metals) are minerals present in living tissues in small amounts. Some of them are known to be nutritionally essential, others may be essential (although the evidence is only suggestive or incomplete), and the remainder are considered to be nonessential. Trace elements function primarily as catalysts in enzyme systems; some metallic ions, such as iron and copper, participate in oxidation-reduction reactions in energy metabolism. Iron, as a constituent of hemoglobin and myoglobin, also plays a vital role in the transport of oxygen.

All trace elements are toxic if consumed at sufficiently high levels for long enough periods. The difference between toxic intakes and optimal intakes to meet physiological needs for essential trace elements is great for some elements but is much smaller for others.

This chapter is a summary of the role of the following essential trace elements in the etiology and prevention of chronic diseases: iron, zinc, fluoride, selenium, copper, chromium, iodine, manganese, and molybdenum. Also discussed are aluminum, cadmium, mercury, arsenic, and lead; these elements have not been demonstrated to be essential for humans but were reviewed by the committee because they are frequently ingested as contaminants in food or water. Interactions between the various trace elements are also briefly considered.

Essential as well as nonessential trace elements have been implicated in the risk of certain chronic diseases in humans, but the evidence is weak in most instances. Some trace elements have been associated with an increased risk of cancer at certain sites, most notably chromium with lung cancer and arsenic with cancers of the lung and skin, but the evidence is based primarily on respiratory rather than dietary exposure. Animal data provide little support for these associations, and no conclusions regarding dietary intake of these elements and cancer risk are warranted at present. In several epidemiologic studies, selenium has been inversely associated with risk of cancer at several different sites, but the data are not entirely consistent and some animal studies do not show this inverse finding. The role of selenium in cancer etiology is unclear. The effects of zinc deficiency on tumor growth are also equivocal; however, zinc deprivation has been shown to alter immunocompetence in experimental animals as well as in humans.

The effects of dietary trace elements on cardiovascular disease risk are not well established. Some epidemiologic studies suggest that copper and chromium may be inversely associated and arsenic directly associated with these diseases or certain of their known risk factors, and some animal evidence supports the findings; however, the data are inconclusive.

Certain other associations of trace elements with chronic diseases have been established with certainty. The ingestion of fluoride in water is clearly associated with a reduction in dental caries. Dietary iodine deficiency is a cause of endemic goiter. Iron deficiency leads to the commonest form of anemia in the United States.

Most other reported relationships between trace elements and chronic diseases are much more weakly supported.

Examples include positive associations of aluminum with Alzheimer's disease and of lead with hypertension.

Calcium

Calcium is the most abundant mineral in the body and makes up 1.9% of the body by weight. Nearly all (99%) of this is in the skeleton. The remainder is in the teeth (0.6%), the soft tissues (0.6%), the plasma (0.03%) and the extracellular fluid (0.06%). Calcium provides a "structural role" in providing rigidity (structure and strength) to the skeleton. This function is provided by a form of calcium phosphate that is generally known as hydroxyapatite [Ca10(OH)2(PO4)6] crystals which are embedded in collagen fibrils (Nordin, 1997).

Calcium ions on the surface of bone can interact with ions in body fluids and act like a large ion exchanger. These properties are important in relation to the role of bone as a reserve of calcium to help maintain a constant concentration of blood calcium (Gurr, 1999). Blood calcium plays an important role to regulate vital body processes such as blood coagulation, muscle contraction, nerve transmission and mediation of some hormonal actions across cell membranes.

Two thirds of bone mass is mineral — principally calcium phosphate — and a healthy adult human body contains 1000-1400 g of calcium, 99% of which is found in the bones and teeth. At birth, an infant's body typically contains 25 to 30 grams of calcium, and the roughly 1000-g difference must come into the body by way of the diet. This much is virtually self-evident. All nutrient intake recommendations for laboratory animals and pets, as well as nonhuman primates, are high in calcium, for purposes of both growth and maintenance.

Humans are at the low end of the calcium intake spectrum. When expressed per unit of energy in the diet, animal calcium intake recommendations are from 3 to 10 times higher than current recommendations for humans.

Calcium serves 2 major functions for bone. First, it is the bulk cation from which bone mineral is constructed. As such, it must be absorbed in sufficient quantity from ingested foods to build a skeleton during growth and to maintain skeletal mass in maturity (the latter by offsetting obligatory losses from the body). Second, it serves as an indirect regulator of skeletal remodeling. The first function has dominated the attention of the clinical nutrition community through most of the past century and provides the foundation for the impressive array of calcium nutritional policy statements referenced above. The second is only now emerging as an important contributor to bone strength.

Calcium as a Source and Sustainer of Bone Mass

There are 2 main physiologic reasons why calcium intake needs to be high: poor absorption and weak conservation. Through most of life, net absorption efficiency for calcium averages only about 10% of intake. The sole exceptions are during infancy, a brief period at the adolescent growth spurt, and during the latter half of pregnancy. Daily obligatory losses through urine and skin average about 200 mg/d in sedentary adults and can be substantially larger under conditions of strenuous exercise. Bone functions as the body's calcium nutrient reserve, and when obligatory losses exceed absorbed intake, bone is destroyed to scavenge its calcium. Unlike sodium, which can be tightly conserved in an acclimated, trained individual, calcium conservation is always poor, probably because of calcium abundance in the foods consumed by evolving hominids. Available evidence indicates that calcium intake of preagricultural humans was substantially higher than were those following the agricultural revolution.

The literature documenting the protective effect of calcium is summarized in the various consensus documents and policy statements cited earlier. In brief, augmenting calcium intake above prevailing levels increases bone gain during growth, reduces bone loss after midlife, and reduces fragility fractures. At last count, there were in excess of 100 metabolic/ physiologic and randomized, controlled trials, more than 90% of which demonstrated the previously cited benefits. In addition, there have been over 145 observational studies, about 80% of which have also been positive.

Thus, there can be no serious doubt about the importance of adequate calcium intake, both to amass the adult skeleton programmed into our genome and to maintain skeletal mass in light of ongoing daily obligatory losses. The question is not whether calcium is important, but rather, how much is enough?

Calcium as a Regulator of Remodeling

Recent work strongly suggests that calcium produces beneficial effects not only through protection of bone mass but through regulation of bone remodeling. The term "remodeling" refers to removal and replacement of small volumes of bone, a process that continues throughout life. Broadly speaking, remodeling of bone serves 2 closely linked purposes: (1) repair of fatigue damage and the reshaping of bone to accommodate growth and altered usage; and (2) as a source and sink for calcium in the protection of extracellular fluid (ECF) [Ca_2+].

In the reconstructive phase of remodeling, bone mineralization takes calcium and phosphorus out of the circulating blood, creating a mineral deficit in the ECF that constitutes the principal systemic stimulus for parathyroid hormone (PTH) secretion. PTH, in turn, is the principal determinant of the quantity of bone resorption occurring throughout the skeleton. In this sense, bone mineralization "pulls" bone resorption. In parathyroidectomized animals and in humans with hypoparathyroidism, total bone remodeling drops to levels less than one sixth the value found in intact organisms. The result, however, is usually hypocalcemia.

During periods of fasting or low calcium intake, PTH secretion rises, and with it, bone resorption (and, thereby, total bone remodeling). From a homeostatic perspective, such remodeling contributes the calcium needed to maintain ECF [Ca_2+]. However, structurally, homeostatic remodeling contributes only weakness, because bone at sites being remodeled is locally reduced in mass and, hence, in strength.

Inadequate intake, poor calcium absorption and excessive calcium losses contribute to reduced mineralization of bone. For example, in rickets and osteomalacia, vitamin D deficiency causes poor absorption of calcium and reduced mineralization of bone resulting in soft, pliable bones that deform easily. A reduction in absorbed calcium causes serum ionized calcium concentration to decline. This stimulates the parathyroid hormone (PTH) that will act in one of three ways to increase and maintain the level of serum calcium. The parathyroid hormone can increase the production of calcitriol (1,25-dihydroxycholecalciferol), which in turn increases calcium absorption through active transport in the gut and tubular reabsorption in the kidneys. Bone resorption may also increase leading to more calcium being released from the bone. Thus, PTH maintains normal circulating calcium concentration during calcium deprivation. It is noted nonetheless, this is done at the expense of skeletal mass.

Low levels of free ionized calcium in the blood (hypocalcaemia) can also result in tetany, which is manifested by intermittent muscle contractions, muscle pain, spasms and numbness in the hands and feet. There is also evidence that implicates low plasma calcium with chronic diseases such as hypertension and colon cancer (IOM, 1997).

Chronic calcium deficiency due to inadequate intake or poor intestinal absorption is one of the causes of reduced bone mass and osteoporosis. Osteoporosis is defined as a skeletal disease characterized by reduced bone mass, increased bone fragility and susceptibility to fracture (WHO, 1994). The clinical and public health impact of osteoporosis stems from its association with fractures of the hip, spine and forearm.

Cooper, Campion & Melton (1992) projected that 50% of all hip fractures in the world will occur in Asia in view of its rapid economic development and rising percentage of the elderly population. If a 20 year old woman consumes 400 mg of calcium a day (half of what is recommended), at age 55, she will have lost 1/3 of her calcium. When your body loses this much calcium, your bones become porous and brittle. They are not as strong, and can break under very little pressure. Women are prone to lose more calcium than men, because of the loss of blood (containing calcium) in menstruation each month. A woman also loses much calcium with each pregnancy. A pregnant mother loses 4 times as much calcium to her baby, as she would in nine menstrual cycles. One of the worst things about osteoporosis is that there really isn't a way to detect it. X-rays only show a decrease in bone mineral content when the loss is at least 60%. Sometimes doctors detect eggshell like bones when they are doing surgery. Patients most often don't even know they have osteoporosis until the condition is serious. Warning signs of osteoporosis include, backache, back muscle spasms, thigh bones aching, difficulty in twisting and bending.

When you don't get enough calcium in your diet, your body takes calcium from your bones and uses it in your body. On some of your long bones (arms and legs) you have rough, crystalline, bumps called trabeculae. (The protrusions you feel on the sides of your knees and elbows are examples of trabeculae.) These trabeculae act as storage sites for calcium and can hold up to 700 mg of the mineral. If your diet is so inadequate in calcium that you don't have much store of it in your trabeculae, then the mineral must be drawn from the more stable bone. This causes osteoporosis.

There is another frightening aspect of a low calcium intake. When your bones don't get enough calcium, they use dangerous heavy metals to fill in the "spaces" not filled by calcium. This can cause cancer. Even if you eat enough calcium, you might not be getting the full benefit from it. Simple carbohydrates from refined white flour and refined white sugar tamper with the hydrochloric acid in your stomach. Your body needs the hydrochloric acid to fully utilize the calcium you eat, so don't eat much white flour and sugar.

If you don't have enough complete proteins in your diet, your body cannot absorb calcium properly. Remember that vitamin D stimulates the production of calcium binding proteins in the digestive tract? Well, if you don't have enough protein in the first place, it can't make the protein transporters needed to absorb calcium.

Your body also can't absorb calcium without balanced amounts of magnesium and phosphorus. (2 parts calcium with 1 part magnesium and 1 part phosphorus.) Magnesium changes calcium to its soluble form so the body can absorb it. Too much phosphorus in the diet takes calcium from the bones and brings it into the rest of the body, making the bones soft. Calcium and magnesium are carried throughout your body by the blood component, albumin. They "compete" for albumin. If there is more calcium than magnesium in the correct ratio, magnesium doesn't get transported in the body to the places it needs to go. This is bad because we don't get much magnesium anyway. This mineral has been lost from the soil as a result of overworking farm land. Your body must also excrete calcium and magnesium in their correct ratio. When there isn't enough magnesium in your body (maybe from too much calcium) your kidneys cannot filter it out because it will make your urine too basic. The calcium binds with oxalic acid or phosphoric acid and is deposited in your kidneys forming kidney stones.

Some particular circumstances can cause your body to lose more calcium than usual. Alcohol is a diuretic and draws out a lot of calcium and magnesium from your body with the increased amount of urine. Just drinking a lot of water can also cause your body to lose more than usual amounts of calcium and magnesium. Exercise and lots of sweating increases calcium and magnesium losses. Calcium is also involved in producing the stress coping hormones produced by the adrenal glands. If you are stressed, then your body will be using some calcium it would normally direct to the bones, in the extra production of hormones. Your bones get stronger when you put pressure on them (walking, weight lifting, running, etc.). If you are immobile, or just don't move that often, your bones will lose calcium.

When you have a lot of calcium in your blood from what you eat, your body releases a hormone (calcitonin) to direct the calcium to your bones. When you don't eat enough calcium, your body has to take it from your bones. Sometimes the body goes overboard and takes too much calcium from your bones. When there is an excess amount of calcium in your blood because of its extraction from bone, your body deals with the problem in a different way. Instead of depositing it in bone, the extra calcium is deposited in damaged organs and arteries. Calcium is a hard mineral, and when it collects in organs and arteries, it causes them to harden also. You can just imagine how well a stiff heart pumps and hard arteries hold up. Arteriosclerosis is a disease that occurs because of hardening of the arteries. It is much harder for the heart to push blood through stiff tubes than soft flexible ones. After time, this will weaken the heart, at which time it can become a target for calcium deposits of its own. A heart with less flexibility having to work harder than it usually would, probably won't function very long. When you consume too much alcohol, fatty deposits accumulate in the liver. This can develop into a disease called cirrhosis. All the fatty deposits hinder the liver's ability to do its job in metabolic processes. Because it is damaged, the liver becomes a good candidate for calcium deposits, which further limits its ability to perform its functions.

Calcium is needed to store glycogen, which is the energy source for muscles. If we could not store glycogen, we would have to eat constantly. Calcium is also important to muscle contractions. When you don't get enough of it, you can suffer painful muscles spasms, like charley horses, especially in the middle of the night. Calcium helps your nerves relax, and is a vital component of the fluid surrounding the brain and spinal cord. The calcium level here is kept constant no matter what is happening to the calcium levels in the rest of your body. Calcium is an ingredient in bile, which helps your body to digest fats.

One of the best ways to get your calcium is through milk and milk products. You can get your daily requirement of 800 mg other ways too.

Calcium bioavailability from foods is of importance when dietary calcium intake is low and when Ca absorptive capacity declines, for example in aging. Low calcium absorption is associated with increased risk of hip fractures in women with low Ca intake (Ensrud et al., 2000). Several factors such as calcium intake, age, estrogen status, vitamin D status, and the intestinal transit time account for part of the individual variability of Ca absorptive capacity. Nonetheless, a large part of the variability remains unexplained. Dietary components that play a role in inhibiting calcium absorption include phytic acid from cereals and pulses, and oxalic acid from some varieties of vegetables. In contrast, dietary components that enhance calcium absorption include lactose and non-digestible polysaccharides (van den Heuval et al., 1999).

Phosphorus is a major structural component of bone in the form of calcium phosphate or hydroxyapatite. The regulation of blood calcium and phosphorus levels is interrelated through the actions of parathyroid hormone (PTH) and vitamin D. A decrease in the blood calcium levels, such as in the case of inadequate calcium intake, leads to a response by calcium-sensing proteins in the parathyroid glands, which secrete PTH. PTH in turn stimulates increased conversion of vitamin D to its biologically active form (calcitriol) in the kidneys. Calcitriol activates the vitamin D-dependent transport system in the small intestine, increasing the absorption of both dietary calcium and phosphorus. Although PTH stimulation results in decreased urinary excretion of calcium, it results in increased urinary excretion of phosphorus. Increased urinary excretion of phosphorus is beneficial because it helps to bring blood calcium levels up to normal, and also because high blood levels of phosphorus suppress the conversion of vitamin D to its active form in the kidneys.

Concerns for phosphorus intake have arisen due to presence of phosphoric acid in soft drinks and phosphate additives in a number of commercially prepared foods (Calvo & Park, 1996). Unlike calcium, phosphorus absorption is not as tightly regulated by the body. Hence, high dietary intake phosphorus gives rise to high blood phosphate levels which in turn, reduce the formation of calcitriol in the kidneys, reduce blood calcium and lead to elevated levels of PTH that may be detrimental on bone mineral content. Abnormally low Ca:P ratio (1:6) has been shown to cause bone loss in animal studies, and there have been reports of excessive fracture rates and low bone density in children with a history of high intake of phosphate-containing coal beverages (Weaver and Heaney,

1999). The concern is also for drinking of soft drinks displacing calcium- containing beverages including milk.

Sodium, Protein and Caffeine Interactions

Sodium intake is an important determinant of calcium excretion because sodium competes with calcium reabsorption in the renal tubules as they share the same transport system in the proximal tubules. (Nordin, 1997). High sodium chloride intake results in increased absorbed sodium, increased urinary soldium and an increased obligatory loss of urinary calcium. Although indirect evidence indicates that dietary sodium chloride has a negative effect on the skeleton, the effect of a change in sodium intake on bone loss and fracture rates has not been reported. Thus, IOM (1997) felt that available evidence does not warrant different calcium intake requirements for individuals according to their salt consumption.

Animal protein has the same effect as sodium as its acid component is able to reduce tubular reabsorption of calcium. It is also likely that animal protein yields sulphate and phosphate residues which tie up calcium as complexes in the renal tubules (Nordin, 1997). It is estimated that for every gram of protein metabolized, urinary excretion of calcium increases by 50% or 0.025 mmol calcium taken out. Nevertheless, while protein intake appear to increase urinary calcium excretion, the effect of protein on calcium retention is controversial. IOM (1997) also pointed out that inadequate protein intakes (34 g/day) have been associated with poor general health and poor recovery from osteoporotic hip fractures. It was thus felt that available evidence does not warrant adjusting calcium intake recommendations based on dietary protein intake.

Caffeine intake in large amounts acutely increases urinary calcium losses in adults and postmenopausal women. While moderate consumption of coffee (1-2 cups a day) had little effect on calcium balance, caffeine may cause a small decrease in calcium absorption. The addition of milk into coffee could ameliorate the adverse effect of caffeine. Available evidence does not warrant different calcium intake recommendations for people with different caffeine intakes.

Calcium levels in the body are very closely controlled so that excessive accumulation in blood or tissues arising from over consumption is unknown. Abnormally high calcium concentrations may occur but usually secondary to diseases such as bone cancer, hyperthyroidism and hyperparathyroidism. The efficiency of calcium absorption decreases with intake, thereby providing the body with a protective mechanism to lessen the chances of calcium intoxication. Currently, the available data on the adverse effects of excessive calcium intake in humans primarily concerns overuse of calcium supplements (National Institute of Health, 1994).

The common effects of excessive calcium intakes are kidney stones (nephrolithiasis), milk-alkali syndrome and interaction of calcium with absorption of other essential minerals such as iron, zinc, magnesium and phosphorous. IOM (1997) had established a tolerable upper level (UL) of 2,500 mg per day for all age groups.

With regards to phosphorus implications, the most serious adverse of abnormally elevated blood levels of phosphate (hyperphosphatemia) is the calcification of non- skeletal tissues most commonly the kidneys. Such calcium phosphate deposition can lead to organ damage. Hyperphosphatemia from dietary cause is a problem mainly in people with kidney failure, since the kidneys are normally efficient at eliminating excess phosphate from the circulation.

Iron

Iron is present in all body cells. As a component of hemoglobin and myoglobin, it functions as a carrier of oxygen in the blood and muscles. Because of iron losses during menstruation, women in their reproductive years require higher iron intakes than men. Therefore, the Recommended Dietary Allowance (RDA) for women 11 to 50 years of age is 18 mg/day, but for men 19 years and older is only 10 mg/day. Women have difficulty achieving this high intake, because they generally have a relatively low caloric intake, and the usual U.S. diet provides only 6 to 7 mg of iron per 1,000 kcal. Since the need for iron is greater during periods of rapid growth, children from infancy through adolescence, as well as pregnant women, may fail to consume sufficient iron to meet their needs.

Iron absorption is affected by many factors. Heme iron is present in meats, poultry, and fish and is more efficiently absorbed than inorganic (nonheme) iron, which is found in plant as well as animal foods. Ascorbic acid facilitates the absorption of nonheme iron, but dietary fiber, phytates, and certain trace elements may diminish it. Food composition data provide no indicators concerning the efficiency with which the body absorbs iron from a given food. The publication Recommended Dietary Allowances (NRC, 1980) provides directions on how to calculate available iron.

The availability of iron in the food supply has increased since 1909, chiefly because of the enrichment of flour and cereal products. The 1977-1978 Nationwide Food Consumption Survey (NFCS) indicates that on the average respondents of both sexes from 1 to 18 years old and females from 19 to 64 years old failed to meet their RDA for iron (USDA, 1984). The Continuing Survey of Food Intakes of Individuals (CSFII) conducted in 1985 and 1986 (USDA, 1987a,b) supports these findings. By itself, however, failure to meet the RDA is not an indicator of poor iron status.

Using data from the National Health and Nutrition Examination Survey (NHANES II), conducted from 1976 to

1980, an expert scientific group of the Federation of American Societies for Experimental Biology (FASEB) assessed iron status (LSRO, 1984a). Five indicators in three different models were used in the assessment. A relatively high prevalence of impaired iron status was found in children 1 to 2 years old, males 11 to 14 years old, and females 25 to 44 years old. Among those whose incomes were below poverty level, impaired iron status was highest in children 1 to 5 years old and females 25 to 54 years old (LSRO, 1984a).

Zinc

Zinc, a constituent of more than 200 enzymes, plays an important role in nucleic acid metabolism, cell replication, tissue repair, and growth through its function in nucleic acid polymerases. These zinc-dependent enzymes include the potentially rate-limiting enzymes involved in DNA synthesis. Zinc also has many recognized and biologically important interactions with hormones and plays a role in production, storage, and secretion of individual hormones. Severe, moderate, and marginal zinc deficiencies have been reported in the United States (Hambidge et al., 1986).

The richest sources of zinc are shellfish (especially oysters), beef, and other red meats. Poultry, eggs, hard cheeses, milk, yogurt, legumes, nuts, and whole-grain cereals are also good sources. Many dietary factors, including other minerals, phytates, and dietary fiber, may adversely affect zinc absorption (Hambidge et al., 1986). Food sources of zinc have changed since the turn of the century. Until the middle 1930s, people obtained about equal amounts of zinc from foods of animal and plant origin, but since 1960, people have obtained approximately 70% of food-supply zinc from animal foods. Zinc from animal sources appears to be better absorbed than that from plant sources.

The 1980 RDA for zinc is 15 mg/day for people 11 years of age and older (NRC, 1980), but zinc available in the food supply amounts to only 12.3 mg per capita (see Table 3-5). Zinc intakes have been estimated in national surveys only since 1984. According to the 1985 NFCS, men and women 19 to 50 years of age consumed an average of 94 and 56% of their RDA, respectively, and children 1 to 5 years of age consumed 73% of their RDA of 10 mg/day (USDA 1986, 1987b).

Data from NHANES II were evaluated by a FASEB group (LSRO, 1984b), which concluded that serum zinc levels are inadequate for assessing the nutritional status of zinc in individuals, but that low values may aid in identifying groups whose zinc status should be further investigated.

Phosphorus

All living organisms require phosphorus to maintain their structure and function. In biologic fluids, it exists as phosphate ion. A major element in hydroxyapatite, phosphorus is a key inorganic constituent of bone. In cells, it is an important part of many life-sustaining compounds, such as phospholipids, phosphoproteins, and nucleic acids; the hormonal second messengers, cyclic adenosine monophosphate, cyclic guanine monophosphate, and inositol polyphosphates; and 2,3- diphosphoglycerate, which is the regulator of oxygen release by hemoglobin. Phosphorus is also the repository of metabolic energy in the form of the high-energy phosphate bond, an allosteric regulator of many enzymes, and an active participant in many physiological buffer systems. Serum concentrations of phosphate serve as one of the regulators of the rate of renal production of 1,25(OH)2D3.

Eighty to eighty five percent of all the phosphorus in your body is in your bones and teeth in the form of calcium phosphate. The 1 1/2 - 2 pounds of phosphorus in your body helps to keep your bones and teeth strong. Phosphorus is important to your bones for another reason. Phosphorus is vital to collagen production and bone is 3/4 collagen. Tendons, ligaments, cartilage, skin, and eyes, are composed greatly of collagen. Without phosphorus, your body could not make any of the above vital connective tissues and organs.

Phosphorus joins up with fatty acids in the body to form phospholipids. Phospholipids have a very interesting characteristic: they are soluble in water and fat. The fatty acid makes phospholipids soluble in fat and the phosphorus makes it soluble in water. This unique trait makes phospholipids very useful as the main component in cell membranes. This allows for fat and water soluble nutrients to pass in and out of the cell. Each cell needs fat and water soluble nutrients to live, so this property is vital. Cell membranes would collapse without phospholipids.

Phospholipids also have a job in the blood. Phospholipids keep blood fat in small globules. Large globules can get stuck on artery walls, which can eventually cause heart disease. Lecithin is a phospholipid used in chocolate to keep it smooth. In the body, phospholipids keep the blood smooth.

Lecithin helps to make bile at an even rate. Bile helps you emulsify fats (break into very small globules). If you don't have enough phosphorus, you can't make lecithin to help make bile, which results in painful gallstones. Lecithin helps to keep fat from accumulating in the liver (cirrhosis).

Phosphorus helps to transport fatty acids throughout your body. It maintains the proper pH in blood and stomach so the needed reactions can take place. Phosphorus has to be present to use fat soluble vitamins A, D, E, and K. Phosphorus combines with carbohydrates to be stored as energy.

Phosphorus is a main component in ATP (adenosine triphosphate), which is the primary source of energy for all living cells. Without ATP, you could not catalyze any reaction. Phosphorus is needed in myelin, which is the fatty covering on nerves to help the impulses travel faster. Phosphorus fatty acid compounds make up 1/3 of the brain's dry weight. Muscles could not contract without phosphorus because the nerves could not properly transmit the impulse without myelin. The muscle would not have the energy to contract without phosphorus containing ATP.

The RDA for phosphorus is identical to that of calcium: 1200 mg until 24 and from then on 800 mg a day.

In a healthy varied diet, we easily get enough phosphorus. Phosphorus is added to processed and refined foods in large quantities. If you eat a lot of processed foods, then you should watch your phosphorus intake so you don't get too much.

You should be careful when eating fresh foods because they could be covered with an arsenic compound containing pesticides. Arsenic and phosphorus are very similar in molecular structure. So similar, in fact, that your body thinks it is phosphorus and puts it in compounds. These compounds of course don't work. This is especially dangerous when you think about phosphorus's role in myelin and cell membranes.

Potassium is a vital nutrient that is in plentiful supply. It is abundant in the fertilizers that have leached out most of the other minerals. Sometimes, though, we don't get enough of it because we need so much in the first place. There is 300 grams of potassium in our bodies. Potassium comprises 5% of the total mineral weight.

Potassium is greatly involved in nourishing every cell in your body. Each cell in the body pulls in nutrients and pushes out waste via the sodium/potassium pump. On the inside of the cell membrane are negatively charged potassium ions (K), and on the outside of the cell membrane are positively charged sodium ions (Na^+). The positive and negative charges are attracted to each other, like in a magnet. The positive sodium ions try to get inside the cell with the negative potassium ions.

If this happened the cell membrane would no longer be electrically polarized, and the pump could not work. This means that most of the poisonous waste products would stay on the inside of the cell and most of the vital nutrients would stay on the outside the cell. Your cells wouldn't live very long if this is what happened. To counteract the results from the natural attraction of K- and Na+, the cell has two protecting mechanisms: first, the cell membrane is strong and doesn't let much Na+ into the cell, and second, the cell membrane is equipped with protein pumps that push the little Na+ that does get into the cell, back outside with the rest of the sodium ions. Because of these mechanisms, K- stays inside of the cell and Na+ stays outside of the cell and the membrane stays electrically polarized. This allows the cell to dispose of its waste products and draw in healthy nutrients.

Nerves also use the K- and Na+ polarization to send nerve impulses. A nerve impulse is much like the "wave" that crowds do at football games. The people in the stands represent the charge directly inside the nerve cell. When the people are sitting down, their charge is negative, when they stand up, their charge is positive. In the nerve, K- lines the inside of the nerve cell, and just as many Na+ line the outside of the cell. When a nerve is stimulated, the first Na+ ion rushes into the cell and the adjacent K- ion rushes out. Once the K- is outside the cell it stimulates the next Na+ to go into the cell, and its adjacent K- exits the cell waiting on exactly the opposite side. As this reaction moves down the cell membrane, the opposite reaction follows it. The first Na+ returns to its place outside the cell, and its K- returns to its place inside the cell. This motion continues along the length of an entire nerve cell. If you're having trouble visualizing it, just think of the "wave".

Muscle contraction is stimulated by nerve impulses. Cramps in the skeletal and digestive muscles have been cured by eating more potassium. Digestive muscles cramping up can cause painful elimination, constipation, and uncomfortable gas. Your heart is a muscle and it too can cramp up. Making sure you eat enough potassium is a good way to keep your heart healthy. Slow and/or irregular heartbeats have been cured by an increase in potassium consumption. A common cause of colic in babies is failure of the digestive system to absorb glucose correctly. This is probably because they don't have enough potassium in their digestive tract for their sodium/potassium pumps to work correctly, and pull in glucose. (It's almost impossible that the imbalance was because of low sodium intake. Baby food is LOADED with salt!)

The sodium/potassium balance is one way the body controls the pH in the body. When the body is too basic they kidneys excrete sodium, and when it is too acidic the kidneys excrete potassium. You can avoid getting kidney stones, by having a more acidic environment in your kidneys. When the urine is too basic, calcium and phosphorus bind together to form kidney stones. By eating a lot of potassium, you will make your urine more acidic.

Sodium and potassium help to keep blood pressure constant. If you don't eat very much potassium, you won't have much in your cells. You're more than likely to have a lot of sodium on the outside of your cells, though. Your cellular pumps have to work extra hard to keep the sodium outside your cell membrane. More sodium will get inside your cells, and with it comes water. Your cells can actually burst because of the amount of water drawn into it. The water comes from surrounding fluids and blood. This causes a decrease in blood pressure. Eating enough potassium will help keep your blood pressure at its most healthful level.

As you can see, potassium's function in the cell membrane has very far reaching effects. Without it, your brain could not transmit messages to other parts of the body and your individual cells would starve to death.

Phosphorus deficiency is very rare by itself. It is usually accompanied by calcium deficiency. As a result, the signs for phosphorus deficiency are almost identical to those of calcium deficiency. Most people get way too much phosphorus, though, so it's not one of those nutrients you can easily be deficient in.

Our bodies need a balanced amount of potassium and sodium so the sodium/potassium pumps in each cell work correctly. Our bodies were designed for diets high in potassium and low in sodium. This was very helpful to our ancestors. For them, salt (sodium chloride, the source of sodium) was a luxury. It was important to eat a lot of salt once they found some, to balance out the great amount of potassium eaten. Because of this need, our bodies are equipped with a salt hunger. (Ever wonder why animals need a salt lick? They eat potassium all day.) Now, when salt is readily available, that salt hunger works against us. Our bodies are rigged not only to want a lot of sodium, but to retain it once we have it. When we eat a lot of potassium, our adrenal glands are stimulated to release aldosterone. This hormone tells the kidneys to excrete potassium and save the sodium. This mechanism has kept the human species alive for thousands of years, but it is killing us. Too much salt causes all kinds of problems.

When a lot of salt gets into your blood, you get high blood pressure. This means that the blood in your body is pushing on the vein wall. It is like trying to run more water through a hose than can comfortably go through it. Your heart eventually stops pumping as hard. The kidneys recognize the drop in amount of blood coming through them and thinks there is a drop in blood pressure. This stimulates rennin and aldosterone to be released. Rennin constricts the blood vessels, which is the last thing you need. Aldosterone directs the kidneys to retain more sodium. When the sodium is drawn back into the body, it brings with it more urea and water. Urea is a toxic poison!

Your kidneys work very hard to keep the delicate sodium/ potassium balance. They filter 325 quarts of blood a day. They were designed to deal with little disturbances in the sodium/ potassium balance. When we overload our bodies with sodium, it is an enormous disturbance. It is hard for the kidneys to get the balance to the correct level. Your kidneys will not function as well, and possibly eventually stop working.

Salt isn't all bad though. If you didn't have any sodium, you would die. Sodium is contained in every bodily fluid. That's why blood, sweat, tears, and urine (don't ask) are all salty. Sodium and chloride help to transport nutrients between cells. Sodium keeps calcium evenly dispersed throughout the blood, so it doesn't collect on artery walls. Salt is needed to produce hydrochloric acid, without which we could not digest our food.

Although a deficiency in salt is hard to do, it can happen. You will experience wrinkles, sunken eyes (because of tissue dehydration), flatulence, diarrhea, nausea, vomiting, confusion, low blood pressure, irritability, and a difficulty in breathing. You probably don't have to worry about it; most of us get way more salt than we need without trying. You need 300-500 mg of sodium a day, and the average American eats 10,000-12,000 mg a day.

Fluoride

Fluoride is an integral part of the food chain. Kumpulainen and Koivistoinen (1977) reported that the measured fluoride content of the diet is three times higher in communities with fluoridated water than in those where the water is not fluoridated. Singer and Ophaug (1979) found that the fluoride content of dry cereals is strongly influenced by the fluoride content of the water in which they were processed. They also reported that baby foods contain high levels of fluoride (Singer and Ophaug, 1979). Fluoride is also consumed unintentionally from two major sources: products containing mechanically boned meat and fluoridated dentifrices. The highest daily average consumption (equivalent to 0.3 mg of fluoride) is reported for children under the age of 5 (Barnhart et al., 1974).

The interaction of fluoride with other dietary ions could influence its bioavailability. Aluminum-containing antacids cause a negative fluoride balance by markedly increasing fluoride excretion (Spencer and Kramer, 1985; Spencer et al., 1981). For infants not drinking fluoridated water, and for those receiving human or cow milk (both low in fluoride) rather than infant formula, fluoride supplements of 0.25 mg/day are advised (Forbes and Woodruff, 1985).

Fluoride could be involved in the growth and maintenance of a normal skeleton (see below and Chapter 23, Osteoporosis). Modest accumulations of fluoride in the bone mineral complex result in increased bone crystallinity and decreased solubility. The net result is the formation of a more stable mineral system that is less susceptible to bone resorption (Spencer and Kramer, 1985).

Selenium

In the 1950s, recognition of the economic importance of selenium deficiency in food animals led to the mapping of selenium distributions in the soils, forages, and blood of humans in several continents. Extreme differences in exposure were found, even within countries. This knowledge enabled investigators to make epidemiologic correlations of diseases in humans and animals and to conduct laboratory experiments to test hypotheses. In 1980, a committee of the National Research Council set the estimated safe and adequate daily intake of selenium at 10 to 40 µg/day for infants, 20 to 200 µg/

day for children, and 50 to 200 μg/ day for those over 11 years of age (NRC, 1980). Studies based on saturation of plasma glutathione peroxidase activity suggest that the selenium requirement of Chinese men is about 40 μg/day (G. Q. Yang et al., 1987). After adjusting for differences in body weight and incorporating a safety factor, a dietary recommendation of 70 and 55 μg/ day can be calculated for North American men and women, respectively (Levander, 1987). The average dietary selenium intake for U.S. men was 108 μg/day between 1974 and mid-1982 (Pennington et al., 1984).

At present, the only well-characterized biochemical function for selenium in mammals is its role in the peroxide-destroying enzyme glutathione peroxidase (Hoekstra, 1975). However, other selenium-containing proteins in mammals have been described (J. G. Yang et al., 1987). Selenium is also known to participate in several important metabolic interactions with a variety of hazardous elements such as mercury, cadmium, and arsenic, which may be important to public health (Levander and Cheng, 1980).

Selenium was named after the mysterious God of the moon, Selene. This mineral is poisonous as it exists in the soil, but plants change it to a form we can use. Selenium is most abundant in soil containing volcanic ash. The soil in northeastern, Pacific, southwestern, and extreme southeastern regions of the U.S. are deficient in selenium. In Canada, the north central and eastern regions are deficient. Food grown in these areas will also be deficient in the mineral. Energy is captured from the food you eat through a process of reactions that go on in every cell. In these reactions, electrons are moved through a process that produces energy. This series of chemical reactions could not take place without enzymes containing or needing selenium. Coenzyme Q requires the presence of selenium to work correctly. Without it, the process would be interrupted and cells would not have energy.

Glutathione peroxidase contains four atoms of selenium, and works as an antioxidant. Sometimes in the energy producing process, molecules can "break", creating dangerous oxidants that ruin your cell membranes. Glutathione peroxidase stops these oxidants before they can do any damage. Without selenium, glutathione peroxidase cannot be produced and your cell membranes could be destroyed.

Selenium also helps to recycle iron from red blood cells. When a red blood cell dies, the iron from that cell bonds to a protein, and forms ferritin. By itself, iron can be filtered out by the kidney, but ferritin is too large to be filtered, thus the iron in it is saved. Transferrin is needed to bind the iron and protein, and selenium helps it to perform this function.

Selenium is a great help to the immune system. It aids in the protection of macrophages, which are large white blood cells who eat viruses, bacteria, and other foreign elements. Selenium helps in the manufacture of interferon, which stops viruses from reproducing. Vitamin A plays a big role in the immune system, and selenium keeps it from being oxidized.

Joints benefit from an adequate intake of selenium. Mucopolysaccharides need selenium to be produced. These molecules lubricate joints and keep them working longer. Without lubrication, the bones in your joints would grind on each other and possibly cause rheumatoid arthritis.

Selenium has the ability to bond with heavy metals in your body. These metals can get inside you from pollution in the air, cigarette smoke, or from the food you eat. When selenium bonds to hazardous metals they can be safely excreted from your body. If they are not excreted, they may damage your organs and even cause cancer.

This may be one reason why scientists believe adequate selenium intake can prevent some cancers. In areas where the soil is deficient in selenium, there is a higher incidence of cancer. Some cancers are caused by free radical oxidation, which selenium prevents. Selenium also encourages the production of macrophages who "eat" foreign material that may cause cancer. It is important to eat foods containing selenium. When foods are processed, all the selenium is destroyed. Once again, if you eat whole natural foods, you will get enough selenium to prevent cancer and rheumatism, and keep your cell membranes healthy.

Men need more selenium that women, because there is a high concentration of selenium in seminal fluid. Adequate selenium may lower the risk of impotence and sterility.

Selenium deficiency is very rare in humans. When the soil has a low selenium content, two diseases occur. Keshan disease affects the health of your heart, and can be prevented by selenium intake. Once you have the disease, selenium supplementation will not help you, as the effects of the disease are permanent. The other disease is Kashin-Beck disease. Characteristics of the disease are swelling and stiffness of the joints in your fingers and arthritis in your elbows, knees, and ankles. This is probably due to the absence of mucopolysaccharides.

Copper

Copper is an essential nutrient that is widely distributed in food and water. In 1980, the National Research Council set the estimated safe and adequate daily dietary intake at 0.5 to 1.0 mg/day for infants, 1.0 to 2.5 mg/day for children, and 2.0 to 3.0 mg/day for those over 11 years of age (NRC, 1980). Pennington et al. (1984) estimated that men consumed a mean of 1.60 mg/day, based on data collected in 1981 and 1982. From data gathered from 1982 to 1984, Pennington et al. (1986) estimated that the mean intakes of 25- to 30-year-old women and men were 0.93 mg/day and 1.24 mg/day, respectively. Intakes of older women and men were lower (0.86 mg/day and 1.17 mg/ day, respectively). In 1985, the CSFII indicated that copper intakes averaged 0.8 mg/day for children 1 to 5 years old and 1.0 mg/day for women 19 to 50 years old, based on 4 nonconsecutive days of intake (USDA, 1987a). The mean intake for men 19 to 50 years old, based on 1 day's intake, was 1.6 mg/day. Schrauzer et al. (1977b) reported copper intakes in 28 countries varying from 1.6 to 3.3 mg/ day.

Cartwright and Wintrobe (1964) estimate that the healthy adult body contains 80 mg of copper. Individual tissues differ greatly in their susceptibility to variations in dietary copper intakes. Subnormal levels of dietary copper are reflected in subnormal blood copper concentrations. Elements such as zinc, cadmium, and iron depress copper absorption and can reduce plasma copper concentrations when ingested at high dietary levels. Copper also plays a key role in iron absorption and mobilization. Elevated plasma copper levels are characteristic of most acute and chronic infections.

Chromium

Chromium is an essential trace element needed for normal carbohydrate metabolism. The biologic function of chromium is closely associated with that of insulin. Most chromium-stimulated reactions are also insulin dependent. For example, chromium functions in carbohydrate and lipid metabolism as a potentiator of insulin action.

Chromium is a trace element found in tiny amounts through out the body. It's main function deals with glucose metabolism. Although it is not well understood, there are some things we do know.

Insulin is a hormone secreted by the pancreas. Insulin moves the glucose in your blood to your cells. This hormone cannot work properly without GTF (glucose tolerance factor). This factor can either be eaten in brewer's yeast or manufactured by your intestines. At the center of this molecule is the chromium atom. Without chromium, you could not produce GTF or insulin. This means that your body would not be able to metabolize glucose or benefit from it. Your brain is mainly nourished on glucose, and without it, you suffer serious mental disturbances. If your body cannot metabolize glucose, your liver cannot make glycogen, which is the energy for your muscles.

Chromium has functions other than the role it plays in GTF. It is a vital ingredient in lecithin, which helps the body keep fat in small particles. When the fat globules get too large, they get stuck on the walls of arteries and can cause atherosclerosis. Your body requires chromium when producing protein. If it can't produce the amount it needs, you can suffer from premature aging. Large amounts of chromium are found in your adrenal glands, indicating its importance in the production of their stress coping hormones. White blood cells contain quite a bit of chromium. When you don't consume enough of the mineral, your white blood cells cannot function properly. This is one of the reasons you are more susceptible to illness when under stress. Chromium activates vitamin C, and is therefore needed to reap the full benefits from it.

It has been difficult to determine the extent and importance of chromium deficiency in humans, partly because analytical techniques are not sufficiently sensitive. Glucose intolerance is usually one of the first signs of chromium deficiency. Among the heavy metals, chromium is the only one whose tissue levels continually decrease throughout life (Schroeder et al., 1962,1970a). The chromium content of diets ranges from 5 to 150 µg/day in the United States to more than 200 µg/day in Japan (Pi-Sunyer and Offenbacher, 1984). The National Research Council (1980) has set 50 to 200 µg/day as a safe and adequate level for adolescents and adults and 10 to 120 µg for infants and children.

The richest sources of chromium include liver and other organ meats, brewer's yeast, whole grains, and nuts. Acidic foods promote chromium leaching from stainless steel cookware, but it has not been determined whether this is a nutritionally useful chromium source (Offenbacher and Pi-Sunyer, 1983). The amount of chromium in foods tends to decrease with processing (Schroeder, 1968). In general, chromium intake is about 50% of the suggested level (Anderson and Kozlovsky, 1985). This is exacerbated by increased chromium losses due to stress (Anderson, 1986). For example, urinary losses of chromium are usually elevated following physical injury and strenuous exercise (Anderson et al., 1982; Borel et al., 1984).

Various forms of stress that affect glucose metabolism often also influence chromium metabolism. At present, it is unclear whether the estimated safe and adequate levels for chromium are unrealistically high.

Chromium content in food, and the amount we need in our bodies, is difficult to measure. You'll need to eat more chromium when you are pregnant because much of it goes to build the baby's store. Most of the time infants are born with high concentrations of trace elements in their bodies. A healthy baby will have enough chromium in their body to last them until age 10. After that the child will need to ingest chromium to uphold their 6 milligram store.

Eating a lot of refined carbohydrates is detrimental to your pancreas and chromium stores. Not only do refined carbohydrates require chromium for metabolism, but they supply no chromium of their own. White rice contains 25% of the chromium found in brown rice. White flour is even worse, containing only 13% of the chromium found in wheat. Replacing complex carbohydrates for refined simple carbohydrates (white flour and sugar) will eventually wear out your chromium supply and possibly cause you diabetes.

Many people are deficient in chromium because they consume too many refined foods. The chromium content in food is hard to measure and can only be estimated. Good sources of the mineral are brewer's yeast, oysters, liver, nuts, potatoes, whole wheat flour, black pepper, and cheeses. It is hard for you to get a toxicity, because your body only absorbs what it needs of the mineral. If you inhale a lot of smoke from coal burning plants or from cigarettes, you run the risk of a chromium toxicity. If you load your body up with chromium from your foods, you can also get a toxicity.

Iodine

Iodine is an essential micronutrient and an integral component of thyroid hormones. In food and water, iodine occurs largely as inorganic iodide and is absorbed from all levels of the gastrointestinal tract.

Dietary deficiency of iodine is associated with enlargement of the thyroid gland and endemic goiter. This is rare in the United States at present, since the mean daily intake is estimated to be much higher than the RDA for all sex and age groups (Fisher and Carr, 1974; Pennington et al., 1986). High intakes are due to the use of iodine in disinfectants, the addition of iodate to dough conditioners, the use of iodophors in the dairy industry, the presence of iodine in alginates, and the use of iodized table salts. No adverse effects are known to result from the present level of iodine in the U.S. diet, but the National Research Council recommends that additional increased intakes should be of concern (NRC, 1980).

Iodine is an essential element in thyroxin. This hormone, along with other iodine containing hormones, controls your carbohydrate and fat metabolism. Without iodine, none of the metabolizing hormones could be produced, and your body wouldn't know what to do with its fuel. You could not grow physically or mentally. In fact, babies who don't have enough iodine suffer from cretinism, a syndrome characterized by spastic diplegia or quadriplegia (paralysis of all four limbs). The infants are sometimes, deaf, mute, have a shuffling gait, and are shorter in stature as adults. Acute deficiencies can affect the infants intellect and neuromuscular ability.

Iodide (not iodine) is pushed into the cells of the thyroid gland via the sodium potassium pump. It moves into the cells 25 times faster using this electrochemical pressure, as it would naturally seep by osmotic pressure. Once inside, the iodide is activated by the protein iodine peroxidase, and can be used to synthesize thyroxin.

Thyroxin not only has a function with metabolism, but with vitamins as well. Carotene from plants cannot be transformed to vitamin A without the help of thyroxin. Vitamin A helps in vision and the immune system. Therefore, if you don't have enough thyroxin, your vision and immune system will both be impaired. Iodine deficiency is what causes most goiters. In some populations, goiters are so common they are considered a normal characteristic. When the thyroid gland doesn't get enough iodine, its tissue degenerates. Massive hemorrhaging occurs in such a large scale that the degenerative tissue gets caught in a pocket of blood. When the thyroid heals itself, brittle, fibrous scar tissue forms instead of healthy thyroxin producing cells. Your body needs just as much thyroxin as it did before, but now it doesn't have as many cells to produce it. To compensate for this loss, the thyroid produces more cells, enlarging your thyroid gland. The enlarged gland is visible on the front of your neck, and known as a goiter. Once you have a goiter, increased iodine won't help it. Remember that the scar tissue is the reason for the enlarged gland, and iodine won't heal scar tissue. It is just about impossible to get an iodine toxicity, as there is a very wide range of safety. Ironically, goiter is also a sign of iodine toxicity. You may also experience chronic fatigue, forgetfulness, lack of interest in sex, impotence, overweight, and irritability.

Manganese

Manganese functions both as a cofactor activating a large number of enzymes that form metal-enzyme complexes and as an integral part of certain metalloenzymes. It is also involved in the metabolism of biogenic amines and participates in the regulation of carbohydrate metabolism (Hurley and Keen, 1987).

Estimates of the human requirement for manganese are based on balance studies. Approximately 0.035 to 0.070 mg/kg body weight per day results in positive balance (McLeod and Robinson, 1972; Schlage and Wortberg, 1972). The daily dietary intake in the United States has been estimated to be between 2 and 4 mg (Kazantzis, 1981). The current safe and adequate intake is 0.5 to 1.0 mg/ day for infants, 1.0 to 3.0 mg/ day for children up to 10 years of age, and 2.5 to 5.0 mg/day for adolescents and adults (NRC, 1980). The best sources of manganese are plant foods, especially cereals, which contain between 10 and 100 mg/kg (Kazantzis, 1981). Manganese toxicity has been observed in humans, but the route of exposure was inhalation in an occupational setting (Ulrich et al., 1979); dietary manganese appears to be nontoxic.

Manganese activates many enzymes and vitamins in your body. It also helps to neutralize poisons in your blood. It helps in the production of such vital hormones as insulin. Manganese also works as an antioxidant to keep your cellular membranes healthy.

Vitamin C cannot work correctly without manganese. Enzymes are needed to direct vitamin C to detoxify the body, fight infection, build collagen, or perform one of its many other functions. Manganese encourages the production of these enzymes, without which vitamin C could not function. In fact, a study done on animals given no manganese showed that when given hydralazine (poison), they died. When manganese was supplemented in the diet and the animals were administered hydralazine, they lived. It is believed to be due to the detoxifying effect of vitamin C, that can only be put to use when there is adequate manganese to activate it.

Manganese activates arginase, which also has a detoxifying function in the body. Ammonia is a substance naturally produced by your body. The only problem is 1/1000 of a milligram of the stuff in a quart of your blood will kill you! Arginase helps to bind ammonia and carbon dioxide to make urea, which is harmless. The urea is filtered out of your blood by the kidneys and excreted as urine.

The specialized beta cells in your pancreas need manganese to manufacture insulin. No manganese, no insulin. Insulin is what moves sugar from your bloodstream to your cells. If you don't get enough manganese, you could get a blood sugar disorder, like diabetes. An observation done on 122 diabetics and an identical control group showed diabetics to be twice as low in manganese than those without the disease.

Manganese activates choline, a phospholipid produced in the liver. Activated choline and ATP form acetyl choline. This compound functions as a neurotransmitter and works in the energy producing Krebs cycle. It also stimulates adrenaline and noradrenaline to be released from the adrenal glands. These hormones help you deal with stress.

Dopamine is a neurotransmitter and needs manganese to be produced. Sufferers of Parkinson's disease have a decreased ability to produce dopamine. Additional manganese may help decrease the effects of the disease. Manganese is needed to produce insulin. When you eat a lot of simple carbohydrates (white flour, white rice, refined sugar) your pancreas has to work overtime to make enough insulin to get the sugar out of your blood and into your cells. Complex carbohydrates (whole wheat flour, brown rice, ect.), on the other hand, do not require so much insulin at one time. It can be secreted at a much slower, steady rate that does not overwork the pancreas.

Magnesium

Magnesium is the fourth most common positively charged ion in the body and is the second most abundant intracellular cation (next to potassium). It plays important roles in osmotic pressure maintenance, enzyme activation, muscular activity, energy metabolism, stabilization of nerve function, and maintenance of bone structure. The average adult body contains about 25 g of magnesium, approximately 50 to 60% of which is found in bone.

Hypomagnesemia results either from decreased intestinal absorption of magnesium or from increased renal excretion. The disease occurs only rarely as an isolated dietary deficiency. It is more often associated with severe general nutritional deficiency, intestinal malabsorption syndromes, excessive vomiting and diarrhea, genetic defects in the kidney, uncontrolled diabetes, and prolonged diuretic therapy. Severe hypomagnesemia (serum levels <1.0 mg/dl) can produce cardiac arrythmias, coronary spasm, hypocalcemia, low blood potassium, changes in mental status, seizures, anorexia, and weakness (Miller, 1985).

Magnesium works to support your bones, helps in the production of cholesterol, helps to activate many vitamins, aids in relaxing muscles, and is an essential factor in protein synthesis.

About 60-65% of the magnesium in your body in contained in the bones. Your bones hold on to magnesium pretty tightly. Even when the rest of your body has a deficiency, your bones will keep most of their magnesium. Only in situations of extreme deficiency will your bones give up their magnesium. Without magnesium, your bones would becomes spongy and could not support the weight of your body. Cholesterol cannot be synthesized without magnesium. Bile, which helps your body digest fats, cannot be produced without cholesterol. Cholesterol is also a vital component of many hormones. Aldosterone is one such hormone, and helps to control the balance of minerals, one of them being magnesium. Aldosterone needs magnesium to be produced and it also regulates magnesium's balance. Cholesterol is also needed in the production of sex hormones, to keep your reproductive system working correctly. The stress coping hormones produced by your adrenal glands also require cholesterol for their synthesis. Cholesterol, along with lecithin and fatty acids (both require magnesium for their formation), are the main components of the myelin lining on the nerves. Myelin protects the nerves from "cross wiring", and helps the nerve impulses to travel faster. Without adequate magnesium to produce these three lipids, your nerves can become ragged and worn out before their time. Magnesium has a calming effect on your nervous system. In fact, when taken in large enough doses, magnesium can have an anesthetizing effect.

Magnesium also has a calming effect on your muscles. Calcium stimulates the muscles to flex, and magnesium relaxes them. Without this relaxing effect, your muscles would cramp up. You may also experience muscle spasms and even convulsions, if you don't get enough magnesium. Remember that your heart is a muscle, and the last thing you want is for it to spasm. Magnesium can prevent painful contractions at the end of pregnancy. It also helps to avoid eclampsia, which is convulsions and coma experienced by the mother after some deliveries.

Magnesium activates vitamins C and E. Therefore, if you don't get enough magnesium, the vitamin C and E that you eat cannot be used, and your body would suffer symptoms of deficiency for those vitamins as well. Magnesium is vital to the production of parathormone, which regulates vitamin D synthesis from cholesterol compounds in your skin. The B complex also requires magnesium for their proper functioning.

Amino acids are the smallest component of protein. Magnesium is needed to properly produce and combine amino acids to make the specific proteins your body needs. Many of the body's hormones, enzymes, and tissues are made of protein. Your body has to produce a lot of each to keep your body running smoothly. The constant repair of your body requires massive amounts of protein to be produced. Without magnesium, your body could not heal itself on the outside or inside. Thousands and thousands of cells in your skin die every day. Much protein is needed to keep it looking firm and beautiful. Your blood is dependent on magnesium to supply it with new proteins, some of which help to kill infectious bacteria and viruses.

DNA is also protein. Without DNA, life would be impossible; it is the instruction book of your cells. We are constantly reproducing DNA in the replication of cells. If we could not produce DNA, we would die in a few days, if not a matter of hours. The replication of DNA allows us to have offspring. Without magnesium, we could not reproduce. Magnesium helps to digest the DNA from the cells in plant or meat foods that we eat.

Molybdenum

The requirement for molybdenum can only be estimated from balance studies (Golden et al., 1985). The estimated safe and adequate intake set by a committee of the National Research Council's Food and Nutrition Board is 0.15 to 0.5 mg for adults (NRC, 1980). High intakes of molybdenum (above 0.5 mg) can compromise copper balance (Nielsen and

Mertz, 1984). Intakes of 10 to 15 mg/ day have been associated with gout in the Soviet Union (Koval'skii et al., 1961). Diet-induced molybdenum deficiency has been found in one patient on total parenteral nutrition (Abumrad et al., 1981). The role of molybdenum in animal and human nutrition has been reviewed by Hainline and Rajagopalan (1983).

Aluminum

Aluminum is the second most plentiful element in the earth's crust. Its concentrations in seawater and freshwater are usually quite low but are increasing in some surface waters because of acid rain.

Ingestion of aluminum in foods ranges from 3 to 5 mg/day (Gorsky et al., 1979; Greger and Baier, 1983). Dietary sources include aluminum used as a filler in pickles and cheese or as a major component of some types of baking powder. Aluminum is also leached from cooking utensils during preparation of acid foods. Drinking water is another source; the U.S. Environmental Protection Agency reported that some municipal waters contain as much as 2 to 4 mg/liter (Miller et al., 1984). Little of the ingested aluminum is actually absorbed, however, so that the total body content is extremely low and does not increase with age (Alfrey, 1986).

Cadmium

Cadmium is known to be toxic at certain levels but may also have a physiological function (Schwarz, 1977). It is absent from the human body at birth and accumulates over the years to approximately 50 years of age (Underwood, 1977). The most recent data from a large-scale survey on the mean cadmium intake from food and water in the United States comes from the Food and Drug Administration's market-basket survey conducted during 1968-1974. These data indicate that the mean cadmium intake from birth to 50 years of age ranges from 26 to 38 μg/day, adjusted for calories and age (Mahaffey et al., 1975; Ryan et al., 1982). Most foodstuffs contain less than 0.05 mg of cadmium per kilogram, but considerably higher amounts may be found in certain types of seafood and in beef liver and kidney (Elinder, 1985).

Cadmium accumulates in the fiber-rich parts of plants and the cotyledon (Moldrup, 1984). The cadmium content of plants varies with the type of plant and soil characteristics, particularly pH. An extensive report on cadmium uptake by plants has been published (CAST, 1980), and the potential hazard of increasing cadmium levels in plants through crop fertilization is being comprehensively evaluated (Bingham, 1979; Ryan et al., 1982; Yost, 1979). In addition to diet, people may be exposed to cadmium through their occupation, household dust, or smoking (Elinder, 1985; Nordberg et al., 1985).

Mercury

In nature, mercury is found mainly in low concentrations as sulfides in the earth's crust, except for rich focal deposits where it may also be present in metallic form. Soil levels of metallic mercury are low (Kazantzis, 1981). Methyl mercury, completely absorbed from the gastrointestinal tract as a lipid-soluble compound, readily accumulates in the brain. Its half-life in the body is estimated to be approximately 70 days (Chisolm, 1985).

Occupational exposure occurs most commonly through inhalation of metallic mercury vapor or of a variety of inorganic mercury compounds such as aerosols and alkyl mercurials. The provisional tolerable weekly intake established by the World Health Organization (WHO, 1972) is 0.3 mg of total mercury, of which not more than 0.2 mg should be present as methyl mercury.

Arsenic

Schwarz (1977) postulated that arsenic is essential for growth in animals, and the evidence for essentiality of very low levels has grown considerably (Anke, 1986; Nielsen, 1982).

Small amounts of this element are widely distributed throughout the soils and waters of the world, and trace amounts occur in foods (especially seafood) and in some meats and vegetables. Arsenic may be present in food as a contaminant (e.g., the unintentional residue of the insecticides calcium arsenate or lead arsenate). Daily intakes of arsenic in the United States are estimated to range from 10 to 130 µg (Buchet et al., 1983).

Absorption, retention, and excretion of arsenic are influenced by the chemical form and the amount in which it is ingested. Rats, unlike other mammals, concentrate arsenic in their blood and appear unique in their metabolic management of arsenic (Dutkiewiez, 1977). Thus, experimental findings from rats may not be applicable to other species.

Lead

Lead is not known to be essential to human nutrition. However, trace amounts of lead (29 ng/g diet) have been reported to be essential in rats to maintain growth, reproduction, and hematopoiesis (Reichlmayr-Lais and Kirchgessner, 1981). Humans are exposed to oxides and salts of lead through various environmental sources, such as automobile exhausts, atmospheric dust, paint, or contaminated drinking water, food, and whiskey. Formerly, the main contributor was the lead that leached into canned foods (Chisolm, 1985), but the food canning industry has since converted from lead-soldered to lead-free cans. At present, the major source of lead exposure is likely to be dust particles from paint or the soil carried into homes.

The World Health Organization/Food and Agriculture Organization (WHO, 1978) recommended a permissible level of lead intake for adults up to 490 µg of lead per day or 7 µg/kg body weight per day. There is no comparable standard for infants and children. In metabolic balance studies, however,

Ziegler et al. (1978) found that a daily lead intake exceeding 5 μg/kg per day is associated with positive lead balance in infants up to 24 months of age. Excess lead intakes by children (blood lead levels >20 μg/dl) have been associated with impairment of a variety of enzymatic and neurophysiological processes (Mahaffey et al., 1982; Otto et al., 1985; Piomelli et al., 1982).

Zinc

Zinc was first recognized as an essential mineral when a deficiency was discovered in young boys living in Iran and Egypt. The symptoms were short stature, anemia, and late sexual maturity. Zinc aids your skeletal growth by helping your body to absorb calcium. Zinc increases the speed at which the hemoglobin in your blood exchanges oxygen and carbon dioxide preventing anemia. Zinc also helps in the production of sex hormones, without which causes late sexual maturity.

The boys mainly ate unleavened bread. The bread is high in zinc, but is also high in phytates, which bond to zinc making an insoluble compound. This made the zinc unavailable to their bodies. When the boys received a zinc supplement, their symptoms disappeared. They grew up to 5 inches in a single year.

Zinc is needed to properly make the hydrochloric acid in your stomach. Without it, you couldn't absorb calcium. This can lead to a calcium deficiency or even osteoporosis.

Anemia is a disease characterized by insufficient amounts of oxygen reaching your cells. This is usually because the hemoglobin in your blood cannot correctly perform its function of transporting oxygen from the lungs to every cell in your body. Hemoglobin not only transports oxygen, but also carbon dioxide. This is a waste product produced by your cells and is carried by hemoglobin to your lungs where it is exhaled. Bicarbonate speeds carbon dioxide in "letting go" of hemoglobin. If carbon dioxide stays bonded to hemoglobin, there would be no room for oxygen to bond to it, and your cells would die as a result of too little oxygen. Zinc helps carbon dioxide to vacate the hemoglobin molecule by working as a coenzyme in regulating the production of bicarbonate. Without zinc, there would be no bicarbonate, and the detachment of carbon dioxide from hemoglobin would be much less efficient. With carbon dioxide stuck to the hemoglobin, there would be no room for oxygen and no way for your cells to get enough oxygen to perform their functions efficiently. Thus, a low intake of zinc, causes less oxygen to reach your cells, and could cause anemia.

Zinc also affects your sexual maturity. It does this in a very strange way though: through your eyes. Light goes through your pupil and hits the cones on the opposite side. Zinc helps the eye to understand that the stimulus it is receiving is light. This stimulus prompts a nerve impulse to be sent from the eye to the hypothalamus in the brain. The hypothalamus stimulates the pituitary to produce hormones, some of them being sex hormones. Without the sex hormones, your body could not mature sexually. Zinc helps to stimulate their production, and therefore, furthers your sexual development. Zinc affects your growth by growth hormones in the same manner.

Zinc must be bonded to insulin in order for it to be stored. It is important to have large amounts of insulin stored and ready to metabolize sugars in your blood. If you had to produce all the insulin you needed in one large effort, you would overwork your pancreas in the attempt, and still not even have enough insulin to metabolize it all. (Actually, this does happen when you eat too many refined carbohydrates which can lead to diabetes.) Zinc helps to store insulin and takes some of the load off the pancreas in its production of the hormone. Insulin also aids in the storage of carbohydrates, which would not be possible without the help of zinc.

Men especially need to eat a good amount of zinc each day, as it is an important to the production of sperm. Quite a bit of zinc is lost with every ejaculation.

If you have been badly burned, zinc can help your skin to heal faster. Your skin needs zinc to heal itself. Your body also excretes large amounts of zinc after a burn. Zinc helps your body to whisk away debris, dead cells, viruses, and bacteria.

During adolescence, pregnancy, postpartum, and menopause the body needs more zinc. Women in any one of these situations should increase their zinc intake.

Zinc deficiency is characterized by short stature, learning disabilities, anemia, and hypogonadism (diminished functioning of the testes). Zinc deficiency also has some of the symptoms of diabetes. Remember the importance of zinc to insulin and carbohydrate metabolism?

Zinc toxicities are extremely rare, as your body excretes what it doesn't need. Most often, zinc toxicities are found in those who have kidney failure and need homodialysis.

Part II

6

Materia Medica of the Bioplasgens

CALCAREA FLUORICUM

Synonyms - Calcii Fluoridum. Calcium Fluoride. Calcarea Fluorata.

Common Name - Fluor Spar. Fluoride of Lime.

Chemical Properties - Formula, Ca F2. Specific gravity of crystals, 3.4. It contains 58.21 parts of calcium. It occurs in nature in mineral Fluorspar; it is beautifully crystalline, crystallizing in various colours and in cubical or octahedral form. It is insoluble in water, but is decomposed by sulphuric acid generating Hydrofluoric acid.

Preparation - Selected pieces of crystal Fluorspar are prepared by trituration, as directed under Class VII, American Pharmacopoeia.

Indications - glandular tumors, varicose veins, prolapsus uterus, bone affections etc.

Facial Signs:

Square folds around the eyes

Diversified folds below the eyes

Brown black coloring around the eyes

Burst veins

Scales, Lines in the face

Cracked lips, corners of mouth, hands, fingers

Periodontosis

Shining skin, Cubicle folds, Single lines which run from the inner corner of the eyes and swoop down below the eyes. The longer and deeper these lines are, the greater the deficiency.

Prominent Wrinkles/Folds below the Eyes

Brown or Black Coloring around the Entire Eye

Broken Capillaries

Scaling or Flaking Skin

Chapped Lips

Periodontitis

Shiny Skin

This salt is indicated in all diseases affecting the substance forming the surface of the bone, the enamel of the teeth and part of elastic fibres, no matter in what structure they may be found. A deficiency of the elastic fibres in the muscular tissue causes a relaxation, which is a primary condition in many diseases.

Indicated in all ailments that can be traced to a relaxed condition of the elastic fibres, including dilatation of blood vessels such as blood-tumors, piles, enlarged and varicose veins, indurated glands, enlargement of the heart, relaxed uvula, prolapsed of the womb, etc. Also useful in the diseases of the respiratory organs with difficult expectoration of small yellow lumps. The symptoms are all worse in damp weather and are relieved by fomentation and by rubbing.

When our body starts becoming less elastic, it could result in hard growths anywhere in the body as well as brittle bones and teeth. Calcium fluoride is the tissue remedy that takes the hard, knotty and brittle out and puts the smoothness back in. There could be no better skin care tips than this. Our skin, our bones, our teeth, our muscles are meant to be in a state of suppleness and smoothness. When there is a lack of this salt is when all the problems related to a lack of elasticity crop up so you can see why it's great for skin care.

Calcium Fluoride is homeopathic potency of Fluoride. Fluoride is an important mineral to help Calcium bond to teeth and bones. Fluoride works by bonding calcium from the saliva to the enamel of the teeth. Calcium fluorica helps with repeated sprains.

Using Calcium Fluoride is so much safer than other forms of Fluoride that are chemical byproducts and actual poisons. Over the counter Fluorides are only to be used topically on teeth, not swallowed. For internal use, use Calcium Fluoride 6X in Cell Salt tablets. Calc Fluor will not cause mottling and darkening of the teeth, which can be a problem in areas that have naturally high amounts of fluoride in the water.

Calcium Fluoride is an important mineral for teeth, skin, bones. It is useful for teething pain and toothaches. Safe for all ages.

If lacking in Calcium Fluoride, emotional symptoms include uncertainty and difficulty making choices.

Symptoms may feel worse in damp weather.

Useful in skin problems such as rough, chapped skin. Colds with green mucous.

Calcium Fluoride is important for tissue strength for varicose veins and muscle tone. Useful for fistulas; hemorrhoids, varicose veins; weak muscle tone.

This substance is found in the surface of the bones, enamel of the teeth, elastic fibers and the skin. A disturbance, or deficiency, in the molecules of this element is shown by lumpy, more or less hard, growths, horny growths, hard crusts with cracked hands, hardened mammary glands, or other parts. Osseous (bone) tumors from injuries, glandular swellings, cataract of the eye, gum boils, displacement or relaxed uterus, sagging abdomen, hardened exudations, hæmorrhoidal knots, varicose veins, and all diseases originating in the elastic fibre and bone covering, which is practically the same thing.

This remedy has proved curative in hard swellings on the bones, varicosis, varicose veins, whitlow, induration of testicles, suppuration, psoriasis, prolapsus uteri, internal piles, ozæna, eczema, knots, gout, defects in enamel, backache, corneal diseases, cataract of the eye, after-pains, bone bruises, catamenia, cough etc., where the above general conditions prevail.

CALCAREA PHOSPHORICUM

Synonyms - Calcii Phosphas Precipitata. Calcis Phosphas. Precipitated Phosphate of Calcium. Calcium Phosphate.

Common Name - Phosphate of Lime.

Chemical Properties - Formula Ca3 (PO4)2.

Dr Hering prepared this by dropping dilute phosphoric acid into lime-water as long as a white precipitate was formed. This was washed with distilled water and dried on a water-bath. Insoluble in water or alcohol, soluble in dilute nitric acid and other acids, and, to a certain extent, in carbonic acid water.

Preparation - The Phosphate of Lime is prepared by trituration, as directed under Class VII, American Pharmacopoeia.

Indications - anaemia, chlorosis, deficient development, dentition disorders, bone affections, dyspepsia, etc.

Facial Signs:

Waxy skin

Skin color like cheese

White coating of the tongue

Halitosis

White noses and auricles

Sweaty hair

Rough voice

A White Coating on the Tongue

The upper surface of the tongue will have a white coating.

Skin Will Appear Waxy

Halitosis [Chronic Bad Breath]

The Nose Will Appear White

The Top of the Head Will Sweat

A Rough and Raspy Voice

The sphere of the Phosphate of Lime includes all bone diseases, whether due to some inherited dyscrasia or to defective nutrition in osseous and other structures dependent upon a proper distribution of lime molecules in the body. It is the bone cell-salt. Without this element, no bone can be formed and hence it is a valuable remedy in childhood when the bones are in the condition of being formed. Cal. Phos. is also found in the gastric juice and plays an important part in the process of digestion and assimilation. It is of importance in anaemia, in chlorosis, in convulsions and spasms, in weak scrofulous subjects; during dentition when the teeth are slow in making their appearance and decay too rapidly; also in other teething disorders. In convalescence after acute and chronic wasting diseases, it acts as a tonic by building up new red blood corpuscles and by restoring the lost vitality. Deficient development of children and young people emaciation without apparent cause onanism, suppuration of bones, spinal weakness and curvature. Aids the union of fractured bones.

Rheumatism of the joints, chronic enlargements of the tonsils and goiter. Cholera infantum, faeces hot and offensive. Dyspepsia; food seems to lie in a lump; vomiting after cold drinks. Cold, change of weather, motion, getting wet, generally aggravates symptoms. Relieved by rest, warmth and by lying down.

It's intake on a regular basis is useful to help with calcium absorption. Important support for growing pains in youth.

Important support for thinning bones during menopause.

Helps solve the problem of hard to dissolve supplements and high Calcium blood levels, but low Calcium levels in the cells.

Calcium Phos is useful in numbness in extremities, painful joints, tooth decay problems.

This element is found in all cells, especially the bone cells, and, therefore, is necessary, in the normal formation of new cells. Its absence, or disturbance, is shown in anæmic states; the weakened conditions following acute diseases; delayed formation of bones in the young; in the knitting of broken bones. Broadly speaking, it is the remedy for weaklings, the ill-nourished, the very young or old, for rickets, chlorosis, open fontanelles, pains accompanied by formication, numbness, cramps, cold sweat, convalescence, convulsions of teething children; stunted children, unhealthy obesity and for the many named and unnamed disease states that have their origin in, and are accompanied by, these general conditions. It has been called the Cell-Wall Salt.

Unhealthy bones of the body and anemia are two of the main problems that follow from a deficiency of this cell salt. In infants, it could be that the fontanelles do not join for a long time and the teeth could make their appearance very late. During teething, children could suffer from a lot of pain, even convulsions. It could take a long time for damaged or broken bones to join together again. With bone growth being slow, children who need this salt and are not given it could stay stunted or have bow legs. In bad cases, it could even affect the spine which could become curved. Children who need this salt could also suffer from crusta lactea or hard crusts on the scalp.

This salt has proved curative in cancer, catarrh, chlorosis, "green sickness," consumption, rickets, curvature of the spine, spinal weakness, open fontanelles, hydrocephalus, bow legs in children, scrofula, albuminuria, anæmia, diseased state of bones, broken bones, convalescence, convulsions, emaciation, painful gums, dentition, headache, leucorrhœa, perspiration (excessive), night-sweats, rheumatism, scrofulous ulcers, clammy feet and hands, tonsils chronically swollen, etc., when the above geneal conditions prevail.

CALCAREA SULPHURICUM

Synonyms - Calcii Sulphas. Calcium Sulphate.

Common Name - Gypsum. Plaster of Paris.

Chemical Properties - Formula, Ca SO4. It is found in nature as anhydrite, gypsum, alabaster and selenite; also in various waters constituting one source of permanent hardness. Molecular wt, 172. It occurs in flattened prisms (selenite) and in earthy masses (gypsum). It is a fine, white crystalline powder, soluble in 400 parts of cold water, insoluble in alcohol and in dilute nitric and hydrochloric acids. It can be obtained by precipitating a solution of calcium chloride with dilute sulphuric acid.

Preparation - By trituration, as directed under Class VII, American Pharmacopoeia.

Indications - suppurations, boils, carbuncles, gonorrhea and chronic catarrhal conditions.

Facial Sign:

Whiteness, alabaster-like skin colouring (like gypsum)

Only few signs in the face

Liver spots

Brown spots

Liver, Sun or Kidney Spots onthe Face These are Brown or yellowish spots around the eyes forehead or cheeks.

A Look of Fatigue

A tired expression on the face. The main functions or purposes of calcium sulfide are to clear the body of heavy metals and in cases of rheumatism. Those who are deficient calcium sulfide will also have an acidic body.

Cradle cap in infants

Adult Acne or Severe Juvenile Acne

Boils or Abscesses [on the Face or Body]

Soft Tooth Enamel

Calcium Sulphate, also called gypsum or Plaster of Paris is a great remedy when the blood in the body is not as pure as it should be. When debris collects in the blood and the cleansing organs in the body cannot perform their tasks well, the impurities in the blood cause infection in various parts of the body. A sufficient amount of Calc Sulph in the body makes sure the blood stays clean and this in turn means the healthy functioning of so many organs.

This is a most excellent remedy in suppurations to which it is closely related. It is an eliminator of effeted matter. A deficiency of this salt causes long protracted suppurations. It is indicated in swelling of the soft parts in connective tissue with threatened suppuration or where suppuration has already taken place. Abscesses either aborting or hastening suppuration. Suppurative stage of eruptive diseases of the skin. Boils, carbuncles, felons, pimples and pustules on the face; suppurative stage of gonorrhea; in fact in all ailments where pus-formations are liable to develop or have already developed. Chronic catarrhal conditions with purulent secretions. Advanced stages of lung diseases.

The true indication for this remedy is a thick, heavy yellow pus, sometimes streaked with blood. Symptoms are aggravated by getting wet or by washing and working in water.

In his later years, Schuessler was inclined to omit this element from his list of "tissue remedies," but the experience of physicians familiar with it is against doing so, for while its sphere is limited, it has been, as stated by Schuessler, "successfully used in many diseases," but he adds, "it does not enter into the constant constitution of the organism," from which it might be inferred that at times other remedies are temporarily useful. Calcarea Sulphurica is useful generally in suppurations, of pus mixed with blood, yellowish discharges from eyes, ears and nose, of this character; boils, carbuncles, wounds, expectoration, pimples, scabs skin diseases, sores, etc., etc. Yellow-coloured suppuration, or discharge, especially if tinged with blood, a general swelling of soft parts threatening pus, or an established vent oozing pus is a call for Calcarea Sulphurica.

Calc Sulph is called for whenever there is pus anywhere in the body tinged with blood. There could be yellow discharges from the eyes and the discharges from the ears and nose are also yellow but tinged with blood. There's a strange thing with Calc Sulph – those who have a deficiency and have a cold will find that the discharge is from the right nostril during the daytime and the left at night. The tongue is usually clay-coloured.

Calc Sulph is also very good at clearing up boils or carbuncles on the back, especially the spine. This needs longer treatment and a dose a day of the right potency for a month often just makes the carbuncle get smaller till it disappears.

A Calc Sulph deficiency will usually be accompanied by thirst and hunger as well as a craving for wine, tea, sour fruits and green vegetables. A person with this deficiency is usually greedy and very irritable and discontented. He is also very ambitious. He feels better when he is warm and his problems are aggravated when he gets wet. Patients who suffer from typhoid fever get better much quicker when Calc Sulph is given along with any other medication that they might be taking.

This salt has proved curative in ear diseases with matter streaked with blood, diarrhœa, boils, abscess, ulcers, carbuncles, festering sores or hurts, pimples, oozing scabs, herpes, catarrh, suppurating glands, etc., when the above-named conditions prevail.

FERRUM PHOSPHORICUM

Synonyms - Ferroso-ferric Phosphate. Ferri Phosphas.

Common Name - Phosphate of Iron.

Chemical Properties - Formula, Fe3 (PO4)2. It is prepared by mixing Nat Phos with sulphate of iron in certain proportions. The resulting precipitate is filtered, washed and dried, and rubbed to a powder, which is bluish-grey from exposure to the air, without odour or taste. Soluble in acids, but insoluble in alcohol or water. It is probably this phosphate which is capable of turning blue, which occurs in the lungs in phthisis in bluish pus and expectorations.

Preparation - The pure phosphate of iron is prepared by trituration, as directed under Class VII, American Pharmacopoeia.

Indications - acute congestions, inflammations, fevers, etc.

Facial Sign:

Reddened forehead, cheeks

Red, hot ears

Red chin

Red tongue

Blue black shade in the nasal root and under the eyes

Grey black colouring around the nose

Pale gums

Full Dark Lower Eyelids

The entire lower eyelid from corner to corner will have a grayish black appearance.

Redness in the Forehead and Cheeks

Red, Hot Ears

Red Tongue

Grayish Black Color around the Nose

Pale Gums

Inconsistent or Light Pigment in the Lips

Iron Phosphate is the salt that is called for at the start of any fever. If given as soon as the fever starts, it can very often bring the temperature down to normal. You usually need doses at very regular intervals – half an hour, maybe even fifteen minutes between doses when the fever is high. What Ferr Phos does essentially is to make sure that oxygen is carried to every part of the body.

Ferrum Phos. is given in the initial stage of all congestions, inflammations and fevers. This salt possesses an affinity or attraction for oxygen and carries it to all parts of the body and hence is an important agent in all diseases in which the blood and the corpuscles are involved. Consequently, the first remedy in all cases depending upon the relaxed condition of the muscular tissue and in abnormal conditions of the corpuscles of the blood themselves. It gives strength to the circular wall of the blood vessels. It supplies the colour to the blood corpuscles. A deficiency of this cell salt is the cause of fevers and inflammatory conditions and so indicated in all febrile disturbances and in inflammatory and congestive diseases at the beginning, especially before exudation has commenced. The principal accompaniments of these conditions calling for Ferrum Phos are manifested by flushed face, fever with full pulse, hot, dry skin, thirst, pain and redness of the part. An excellent remedy in anaemia, chlorosis, pneumonia, inflammatory rheumatism, tonsillitis, diphtheria, cystitis, nosebleed, incontinence of urine, apoplexy, gastritis etc. The symptoms calling for this remedy are always aggravated by motion and ameliorated by cold.

This element is contained in the red blood corpuscles and possesses "the property of attracting oxygen" from the inhaled air. Any disturbance in this salt is shown primarily by relaxed muscular tissue with inflammation, fever, heat, congestion, throbbing, swelling, with the innumerable succeeding ills. From its character Ferrum Phosphoricum is necessarily almost always the first remedy required in every attack of acute illness. It is the first in every itis, from bronchitis on through the list to tonsillitis. It is of the blood and is, as Rademacher said, a "universal remedy." It precedes and then the other remedies follow in acute ills. In longseated ills, this remedy does not always hold true. It is also required in some anæmic conditions and those following loss of blood.

When the red blood corpuscles of the blood are made stronger, it means the body can be better oxygenated and this in turn means any attack can be better repulsed and any weakness better attended to. Ferr Phos is rarely prescribed for ailments that are chronic or long standing. It is of great help in the first stages of any 'itis' – be it laryngitis, bronchitis or tonsillitis. It also helps when there is a sudden earache that comes on, a sudden fever, nosebleed or sprain. You can progress to other tissue remedies after a dose of Ferr Phos has been given. It stops any internal bleeding and prevents inflammation. A patient who needs Ferr Phos usually has a red, flushed face.

A deficiency of Ferr Phos is one of the main causes for anemia. When there is sufficient Ferr Phos in the system, there is a better metabolization and absorption of iron. It's a great tonic for women during their periods when the loss of blood makes them feel tired and run down. People who lack Ferr Phos usually have a craving for coffee and don't like milk.

This remedy has proved curative in bronchitis, gastritis, laryngitis, mastitis, nephritis, pericarditis, periostitis, phlebitis, pleuritis, tonsillitis, as a primary remedy; abscess, rheumatism, hæmorrhages (red blood), boils, catarrhal colds, congestions, inflammations, coughs, croup, deafness, diarrhœa, earache, erysipelas, swellings, gonorrhœa, gum-boils, hæmorrhoids, nose-bleed, fever, headache irritations, neuralgia, palpitation, pleurisy, quinsy, scarlet fever, sprains, wounds, etc. when the indications noted above are in evidence.

KALI MURIATICUM

Synonyms - Potassium Chloride. Kali Chloratum. Kali Chloridum. Potassii Chloridum.

Common Names - Chloride of Potash or Chloride of Potassium. (N. B - This drag must not be confounded with Kali Chloricum, whose synonyms are Potassium, Chlorate, Potassae Chloras and Potash Chloras, whose common name is Chlorate of Potash, and whose formula is K CI O3. This has been proved, and the authors of the "Guiding Symptoms" have deemed them sufficiently similar to Schuessler's Kali Mur to incorporate them in their work. See Vol. VI, "Guiding Symptoms")

Chemical Properties - Formula, K Cl. Occurs in nature in mineral carnallite. It may be prepared by neutralizing pure aqueous hydrochloric acid with pure potassium carbonate or hydrate. It crystallizes in cubes, occasionally in octahedrons. The crystals are colourless or white, melt at a low red heat and volatilize at a high temperature without decomposition. It is soluble in three parts of cold and two of boiling water, and is insoluble in strong alcohol.

Preparation - The pure chloride is prepared by trituration, as directed under Class VII, American Pharmacopoeia.

Indications - second stage of inflammatory diseases, diphtheria, croup, catarrh, pneumonia, glandular swellings, deafness etc.

Facial signs:

Milky skin

Blue white skin colour

Skin like cheese

Swollen lymphatic knots

White coating of the tongue

Mealy skin dandruff

Stuck together eyes

Squinting, As If Light-Sensitive. Those are the potassium chloride deficiency will squint as though the light is bothering their eyes.

Milky White Skin [Also Present in Vitamin D Deficiency]

Swollen Lymphatic Knots

White Coating on the Tongue [Also See Calcium Phosphate]

Flaking of the Skin

Any discharge that is white or grayish-white calls for Kali Muriticum or potassium chloride. This indicates the second stage of congestion – whether in the nose, throat or lungs. The first stage is usually a clear, watery discharge and the third stage is a yellowish discharge. This salt is very useful for congestion in the chest, particularly for congestion in infants. Among the tissue salts, it's one of the primary congestion remedies. Kali Muriticum is essential in the formation of fibrin in the blood and when there is a lack of it, a white discharge is the result.

Kali Mur. is given for the sequel of all inflammations, for exudations and infiltrations, especially of a fibrous character and in inflammations of serous membranes, when the exudation is plastic in nature. A most excellent remedy in the later stages of all catarrhal states. This cell-salt works with the fibrine, which is found in every tissue of the organism except boric. In inflammatory exudations we find fibrine in the serous cavities and on the mucous membranes. The use of Kali Mur. usually follows Ferrum Phos. in inflammatory disorders. The characteristic symptoms of Kali Mur which is always indicated in the second stage of the inflammatory diseases, are glandular swellings, discharges or expectorations of a thick, white fibrinous consistency, white or gray exudations and a white or gray coating of the tongue. The efficacy of this remedy is demonstrated in chronic catarrhal conditions, croup, diphtheria, dysentery, pneumonia etc. Diarrhoea with pale, yellow faces. With Ferrum Phos is should be given in coughs. Useful in deafness from the catarrh of the Eustachian tubes, in skin eruptions with small vesicles containing yellowish secretions, ulcerations, ulcerations with swelling and white exudations, in rheumatism with swelling of the parts, in leucorrhoea and gonorrhea with characteristic discharge. Symptoms in general are worse from motion, while gastric and abdominal symptoms are worse after taking pastry, rich and fatty foods.

This element, or salt, is chemically related to fibrine. Like Ferrum Phosphoricum, it is found in almost all cells. "It will dissolve white, or grayish-white, secretions of the mucous membranes and plastic exudations," consequently it is called for in catarrh, croupous, and all plastic exudations of mucous membranes that are white or grayish-white. It almost always follows Ferrum Phosphoricum for the secondary conditions or states succeeding inflammation. It is indicated in the white or grayish, coated tongues, in catarrh and diseases showing that peculiar colour of the exudations of the mucous membranes. It is especially useful in ear diseases, catarrh of the middle ear and closed Eustachian tubes, cracking noises, deafness, etc.; coughs, hoarseness and bronchial troubles; sluggish liver, light- coloured stools, lung diseases showing characteristic coloured expectoration. Like Ferrum Phosphoricum, it is a useful inter-current remedy in many cases.

This salt has proved curative in abscess, adhesions, rheumastism, asthma, bronchitis, congestions, "colds," catarrh, coryza, constipation, cough, croup, deafness and ear diseases, chancre, diarrhœa, diphtheria, dropsy, dyspepsia, eruptions, exudations, excoriations, gastritis, gonorrhœa, hæmorrhage of dark, clotty blood (Ferr. Phos., bright blood), headache, hoarseness, whooping cough, indigestion, liver diseases, lung diseases, measles, meningitis, menstruation, mumps, orchitis, pimples, pleurisy, childbirth fever, fevers secondary stage, pains rheumatic, scarlet fever, sick headache, stomach derangements, swellings without fever, sycosis, throat diseases, quinsy, mucous ulcerations, vomiting dark blood, diseases of mucous membranes, etc., when the above-named conditions in general prevailed.

Kali Muriticum is an excellent remedy in the early stages of deafness when it is caused because of a blockage of the Eustachian tubes. This could be due to an infection or due to mucous blocking the tubes. It also helps lessen the pain of an earache which comes on due to exposure or changes in atmospheric pressure. Taken at the right time, it also clears out the sinuses and gets rid of a sick headache that comes on with a cold.

Kali Muriticum is the second line of attack in any fever and it is very often used with Ferr Phos to fight a fever and bring the temperature down. It is also very helpful to relieve the pain of rheumatism.

Kali Muriticum is a great remedy for the skin too. It helps when the skin gets very dry and there are dry, white, scaly discharges from the skin. It is of great benefit in children's eczema especially when it affects the face. The low potencies, when dissolved in water make an excellent first aid remedy for burns and blisters. It is a great 'healing' remedy and helps wounds stop bleeding and heal faster.

For second stage of inflammatory diseases, diphtheria, croup, catarrh, pneumonia, glandular swellings, deafness etc.

Kali Muriticum is given for the sequel of all inflammations, for exudations and infiltrations, especially of a fibrous character and in inflammations of serous membranes, when the exudation is plastic in nature. A most excellent remedy in the later stages of all catarrhal states. This cell-salt works with the fibrine, which is found in every tissue of the organism except boric. In inflammatory exudations we find fibrine in the serous cavities and on the mucous membranes. The use of Kali Mur. usually follows Ferrum Phos. in inflammatory disorders. The characteristic symptoms of Kali Mur which is always indicated in the second stage of the inflammatory diseases, are glandular swellings, discharges or expectorations of a thick, white fibrinous consistency, white or gray exudations and a white or gray coating of the tongue. The efficacy of this remedy is demonstrated in chronic catarrhal conditions, croup, diphtheria, dysentery, pneumonia etc. Diarrhoea with pale, yellow faces. With Ferrum Phos is should be given in coughs. Useful in deafness from the catarrh of the Eustachian tubes, in skin eruptions with small vesicles containing yellowish secretions, ulcerations, ulcerations with swelling and white exudations, in rheumatism with swelling of the parts, in leucorrhoea and gonorrhea with characteristic discharge. Symptoms in general are worse from motion, while gastric and abdominal symptoms are worse after taking pastry, rich and fatty foods.

KALI PHOSPHORICUM

Synonyms - Potassium Phosphate. Potassii Phosphas.

Common Name - Phosphate of Potash.

Chemical Properties - Formula, K2 H P O4. Prepared by mixing aqueous phosphoric acid with a sufficient quantity of potash, hydrate or carbonate, until the reaction is slightly alkaline, and evaporating. It crystallizes with difficulty. It is very deliquescent; it is freely soluble in water and insoluble in alcohol.

Preparation - It is prepared by trituration, as directed under Class VII, American Pharmacopoeia.

Indications - neurasthenic condition in general, sleeplessness.

Facial Signs:

Ash-grey skin, mainly in the chin area

Grey ocular part

Sunken temples

Absent expression

Brown coating of the tongue

Dry tongue

Periodontosis

Gum bleeding

Halitosis

Sunken Temples

Look for indents just beyond the outside corner of the eyes.

Grayish Skin, Mainly in the Chin Area

Gray Eyes

Absent Expression

Brown Coating on the Tongue

Dry Tongue

Periodontitis

Bleeding Gums

Halitosis [Chronic Bad Breath]

Kali Phos. is a constituent of the brain, nerves, muscles and blood vessels. It unites with albumen and creates nerve fluid or the gray matter of the brain. Nervous symptoms indicate a deficiency of this cell- salt, which must be supplied to restore the normal condition. Whatever disease can be traced to the nerve degeneracy, we enter the field of Kali Phos. Nervous condition known as neurasthenia is a field in which this salt has become prominently curative. The results of the want of nerve power, such as prostration, loss of mental vigor, depression, brain-fag, softening of the brain, insanity, paralysis, epilepsy, hysteria, locomotor ataxia and when there is rapid decomposition of the blood. It is curative in septic haemorrhages, scorbutus, gangrene, stomatitis, offensive carrion-like diarrhoea, dysentery, a dynamic or typhoid conditions, incontinence of urine, urticaria, predisposition of epistaxis in children, dizziness and vertigo from sleeplessness, nervous exhaustion, nervous dyspepsia, asthma, neuralgia, nervous headaches, tongue coated as if with dark liquid mustard. Symptoms are aggravated from noise, by mental or physical exertion, by rising from a sitting position. Pains worse in cold and ameliorated by gentle motion.

This is the chief "nerve salt," and is found in the brain cells, and nerve fluids, the blood plasma (white corpuscles) and the inter-cellular fluids. A disturbance, or deficiency, in the normal state of this physiological element shows, mentally, in despondency, anxiety, fearfulness, weak memory, mental decay, mental and physical break-down, neurasthenia, hypochondria, hysteria, insomnia, night terrors, irritability, insanity and paralysis; also in septic conditions, typhus, scurvy, ulcerations and physically degenerated states, generally, foul states and discharges, gangrene, blackish, thin blood, putrid conditions. Decay generally, mental and physical.

This salt has proved curative in nervousness, neurasthenia, anxiety, gloom, morbidness, depression, brain-fag, loss of memory, sleeplessness, delirium tremens, horrors, dread, epileptic fits, hypochondria, hysterias, insanity, nervous diseases, paralysis, night terrors, palpitations, exhaustion, softening of the brain, sexual weakness, septic states, typhus, typhoid, gangrene, black small-pox, appendicitis, amenorrhœa, asthma, blood blackish but thin, Bright's disease, cancer, chancre, cholera, croup, cystitis, deafness, diabetes, diarrhœa, dysentery, diphtheria, eczema, epilepsy, nose-bleed, headache, hæmorrhage blackish and thin, rickets, putrid sore throat, sciatica, sepsis, spinal diseases, suppurations foul, etc. when the above-named conditions are present.

What does Kali Phosphoricum do that makes it act in two very opposite ways where the brain is concerned? All it does is to make sure the brain performs to its full capacity and as it ought to. Which means, stay active when it should and get its well deserved rest when it should. Kali Phosphoricum is a great nerve tonic and it brings the brain back to its state of equilibrium.

There are physical, mental and emotional symptoms that call for the tissue salt Kali Phosphoricum is the remedy for brain fag or nervous exhaustion. Anyone who has to use his mental capabilities a lot and feels drained out at the end of the day needs Kali Phosphoricum to help him cope. Without this tissue remedy, there could be many symptoms that are manifested – from a failing memory to anxiety, depression, hysteria and even insanity. It helps a lot for people prone to nightmares.

Kali Phosphoricum gives relief in cases of gangrene as well as septic conditions. It also alleviates the pain of sciatica and cancer. Bad breath and receding gums get better with Kali Phosphoricum. Taken for a few days before traveling, it helps to keep you fresh with hardly any jet lag so it's great for businessmen who have to travel a lot and suffer from the ill effects of various time zones.

The results of the want of nerve power, such as prostration, loss of mental vigor, depression, brain-fag, softening of the brain, insanity, paralysis, epilepsy, hysteria, locomotor ataxia and when there is rapid decomposition of the blood. It is curative in septic haemorrhages, scorbutus, gangrene, stomatitis, offensive carrion-like diarrhoea, dysentery, a dynamic or typhoid conditions, incontinence of urine, urticaria, predisposition of epistaxis in children, dizziness and vertigo from sleeplessness, nervous exhaustion, nervous dyspepsia, asthma, neuralgia, nervous headaches, tongue coated as if with dark liquid mustard. Symptoms are aggravated from noise, by mental or physical exertion, by rising from a sitting position. Pains worse in cold and ameliorated by gentle motion.

KALI SULPHURICUM

Synonyms - Potassium Sulphate. Kali Sulphas. Potassae Sulphas. Potassii Sulphas.

Common Name - Sulphate of Potash.

Chemical Properties - Formula, K SO 4. Occurs native in lavas, etc. Crystallizes in short, permanent, colourless four and six-sided prisms. It is soluble in ten parts of cold and three parts of boiling water. It is insoluble in alcohol. It has a sharp, bitter, saline taste.

Preparation - Pure sulphate of potash is prepared by trituration, as directed under Class VII, American Pharmacopoeia.

Indications - third stage of inflammatory or catarrhal condition, leucorrhoea, diarrhoea, skin diseases, rheumatism, ulcerations, dyspepsia.

Facial Signs:

Brown-yellow skin

Dark eyelids

`Yellowish around the mouth

Freckles

Dandruff on viscous base

Sticking head dandruff

Yellow and slimy coating of the tongue

Dark Eyelids

The entire upper eyelid will be dark in color.

Yellowish–Brown Skin

Sun Induced Freckles on the Skin

Dandruff Which Sticks to the Head

Yellow, Slimy Coating on the Tongue

A clear skin needs a lot of work inside the body and one of the best ways to ensure your skin is clear is by making sure your blood and through it your body stays well oxygenated. Potassium sulphate is the salt that makes sure the oxygen you inhale gets transferred into the cells. While Ferr Phos makes sure it gets to the places where the oxygen is needed, it is Kali Sulphuricum that makes the transfer effective.

Kali Sulph is a carrier of oxygen. It furnishes vitality to the epithelial tissues. Light yellow, sticky and watery secretions are the characteristics of this remedy. The chief indication for this remedy is yellow deposit on the tongue. It has been given in bronchitis with yellow, slimy or thin, watery expectoration, in whooping cough, pneumonia pthisis, skin diseases with a sticky yellowish secretion and peeling off of the epidermis. Epithelioma, rheumatism, retrocession of eruptions in measles. Dyspepsia with slimy yellow coating of the tongue, catarrh of the bowels, diarrhoea, leucorrhoea, ophthalmia etc; with light yellow, watery secretions; dandruff; yellow scales in skin diseases. Amenorrhoea, menstruation too late and too scanty with weight and fullness in the abdomen etc. All ailments are worse in a warm room and toward evening and better in cool, open air.

This salt is essentially a 'skin' remedy and a lack of it can cause dull, sickly skin. When there's enough of the salt in the body, that's all the clear skin tips you need because the skin shows it – clear and glowing. This salt should be present in the right quantities in the epidermis of the skin in order to keep it clear and free from blemishes.

Kali Sulphuricum is an excellent remedy for conjunctivitis or sore eyes when the discharge is yellow. When a person has a bad cold and loses all sense of smell, Kali Sulphuricum uricum will help. The skin could have eruptions like eczema or dandruff but you'll recognize the Kali Sulphuricum uricum skin ailments because they will be scaly and yellow.

A lack of this salt will usually result in loose motions and a constant feeling of being full. There could also be a burning sensation in the stomach. Women go through scanty periods which come late and suffer from heaviness in the abdomen. Many suffer from shifting rheumatic pains that run through the body and the legs hurt at night.

A deficiency of this salt shows up in a very fast pulse. The person drops off to sleep, then wakes up with a start because he has had a nightmare. He could suffer from dizzy spells and vertigo and is usually very shy and timid, yet jealous and suspicious. His moods keep changing without any reason.

For third stage of inflammatory or catarrhal condition, leucorrhoea, diarrhoea, skin diseases, rheumatism, ulcerations, dyspepsia.

Like Ferrum Phos. This salt aids in effecting the transfer of the inhaled oxygen. It is found in nearly all the cells containing iron. Any abnormality or deficiency is shown physically, by a sensation of weariness and heaviness, with chilliness, headache, pains in the limbs, or vertigo. The malaise is worse when patient is confined in rooms, and from warmth and is better in the open, or in cool, air. It is called for in desquamation following diseases like scarlet fever, measles, etc., scaly skin, yellowish eczemas, dandruff, etc. It is indicated in conditions of the mucous membranes, exudations, discharges, secretions and tongue, when the colour is distinctly yellow or yellowish.

Has been successfully prescribed in bronchitis, catarrh, albuminuria, diphtheria, dropsy, vertigo, asthma, ear diseases, whooping cough, syphilis, tuberculosis, stomach catarrh, anæmia, rheumatism, opthalmia, lupus, eczema, skin diseases, measles, menstruation, leucorrhœa, indigestion, diarrhœa, disorders of the eye, etc., when general characteristics and general indications as above are shown.

MAGNESIA PHOSPHORICUM

Synonyms - Magnesium Phosphoricum.

Common Name - Phosphate of Magnesia.

Chemical Properties - Formula, Mg HPO 4, 7H2O. It is made by mixing phosphate of soda with sulphate of magnesia. The crystals resulting are six-sided, needle-like. They have a cooling, sweetish taste. They are sparingly soluble in water; 322 parts dissolving one part after standing a long time. Boiling decomposes it. It exists in the grains of cereals, and can be detected in considerable quantity in beer.

Preparation - The salt is triturated according to Class VII, American Pharmacopoeia.

Indications - convulsions, epilepsy, cramps and spasmodic affections, neuralgia, sciatica.

Facial Sign:

Red, round spots on the cheeks (always or temporarily)

Red spots in the neck

Otherwise pale skin

Convulsions of the corners of mouth

Twitch of the eyelids

Red Spots

Look for red spots on the cheeks or neck.

Other Facial Signs to Help Confirm the Deficiency:

Otherwise Pale Skin

Convulsions in the Corners of the Mouth/Lips

Twitching of the Eyes

Magnesium Phosphoricum is also very useful in infants' colic where three or four doses that are given at intervals of ten minutes bring about immense relief to a suffering baby.

Magnesium Phosphoricum also relieves the pain of a sudden toothache or a sudden headache with shooting pains. The pain that calls for Magnesium Phosphoricum is sudden and lightning-like. Any dull ache needs another remedy. Where Magnesium Phosphoricum has proved of immense use is during labor where it eases the pain and facilitates an easy delivery.

This tissue remedy has also been used in cases of paralysis in the early stages with a lot of success. It is also used to ease the intensity of an epilepsy attack where the liquid is used to moisten the tongue of the patient in case the pills go down the wrong way and cause choking.

For convulsions, epilepsy, cramps and spasmodic affections, neuralgia, sciatica.

It is a constituent of muscles, nerves, brain, bone, spine, teeth and blood corpuscles. It helps to create the white fibres of the muscles and nerves. It uses water and albumen to form the transparent fluid, which nourishes the white threads and fibres of nerves and muscles. The deficiency of this salt allows the fibres to contract, causing spasms, cramps, convulsions and other nervous phenomena. It is a remedy to be thought of in all maladies having their origin in nerve cells and in the muscular tissue. It is particularly indicated in lean, thin, emaciated persons of a highly nervous temperament. Magnesia patient is always languid, tired and easily exhausted. The value of this remedy is shown in all forms of spasms, cramps, tetanus. St. Vitu's dance, epilepsy, spasmodic retention of urine, paralysis agitans, hiccup, whooping cough, chorea. It is the remedy for the neuralgic pains in the head, face, teeth, car, stomach, abdomen etc. spasmodic palpitation of the heart, dysmenorrhoea. Attacks are often attended with great prostration, sometimes with profuse sweat. Valuable remedy for flatulent colic forcing the patient to bend double. Dysentery with cramp-like pains, angina pectoris, sciatica with excruciating spasmodic pains, angina pectoris, sciatica with excruciating spasmodic pain writer's and piano-player's cramps. All pains are lightening-like, shooting or boring, and change their location frequently and are worse on the right side, from cold air, washing in cold water, and from touch. Relieved by warmth pressure, friction and by bending double.

This salt, or element, is found in the blood-cells, muscles, brain, spinal marrow, nerves, bones and teeth. A disturbance, or deficiency, of it is shown in sharp pain, cramps and paralysis. The patient is better from warmth and gentle but from pressure, but worse from a light touch or jar. Its diseases take the form of neuralgia, toothache, faceache, convulsions, fits, cramps, colics, spasms, palsy, trembling, twitching, hiccough, tetanus and similar conditions. Its pains are likely to be of a lightning like character. It is the opposite to the other great nerve remedy, Kali Phos., which betokens degeneration and decay, while Mag. Phos. is generally evidenced by acute pain.

It has been successfully prescribed in neuralgia, sharp pain, cramps, agina pectoris, chorea, St. Vitus's dance, epilepsy, colic, convulsions, cough, whooping cough, diplopia, dysentery, faceache, toothache, labour pains, menstrual colic, colic, ovarian neuralgia, puerperal convulsions, laryngismus stridulus, palsy, spasmodic retention of urine, spasmodic conditions, stricture, squinting, teething, tetanus, trembling, etc., when general conditions indicate a deficiency of this salt, as noted above

NATRUM MURIATICUM

Synonyms - Sodium Chloride. Chloruretum Sodicum. Natrium Chloratum Purum. Sodii Chloridum. Chloride of Sodium.

Common Names - Common Salt. Table Salt.

Chemical Properties - Formula, Na Cl. It occurs abundantly in nature, nearly everywhere. It crystallizes from aqueous solutions in colourless, transparent, anhydrous cubes; it is soluble in three parts of cold water, scarcely more in boiling. It is insoluble in absolute alcohol. Its watery solutions dissolve several bodies insoluble in water, e. g, Calc Phos etc.

Preparation - One part of weight of pure chloride of sodium is dissolved in nine parts by weight of distilled water. Amount of drug power, one-tenth. Dilutions must be prepared according to Hahnemann's methods.

Indications - catarrhal affections with thin, clear, transparent, watery secretions, influenza, hay-fever, diarrhoea, constipation, leucorrhoea, intermittent fevers and skin diseases.

Facial signs:

Humid shine on the upper eyelid, like snail mucus (gelatin shine)

Bright eyelids

Big skin pores

Bloated face, eye puffiness, spongy cheeks

Swollen, spongy cheeks, deep nasolabial folds

Head dandruff

White seclusions of the eyes

Clear coating of the tongue

Salivary vesicles on the edge of the tongue

Skin rash in the upper forehead

Itch

Dry skin

Deep Naso-labial Fold

These are the lines that run from the corners of the nose, where the nose flares and run down the outside corners of the lips. If these lines are present and are deep, this is the strongest indication that the individual is deficient in sodium chloride.

Shiny Upper Eyelids [Almost Wet Appearance]

Bright Upper Eyelids [Reddish]

Bloated or Puffy Face

Dandruff

Clear Mucus like Coating on the Tongue

Silver Stripe below the Eyelashes

Swollen Taste Buds

Rash on the Upper Forehead

Itchy/Dry Skin

This salt is a constituent of every liquid and solid part of the body. Its function is to regulate the degree of moisture within the cells. It properly distributes the water through the organism.

Deficiency in this salt causes the disturbance of water in the human organism. An unequal distribution of water in the system sometimes causes excessive dryness of mucous membranes in some part, while there may be a copious, watery fluid from another part. Natrum Mur. will set things right and will establish equilibrium. It acts upon the lymphatic system, the blood, liver, spleen and upon the mucous lining of' the alimentary canal. It is indicated in headache, toothache, faceache, stomachache and also where there is either salivation or hyper secretion of tears or vomiting of water and mucus. Catarrhal affections of mucous membranes with secretion of transparent, watery, frothy mucus. Small watery blisters, breaking and leaving a thin crust. Skin diseases with watery symptoms. Diarrhoea with transparent, frothy, slimy stools. Constipation with dull headache and profuse tears.

Conjunctivitis with clear watery discharge. Tongue clean, slimy, small bubbles of frothy saliva on sides. Leucorrhoea with watery, smarting or clear, starch-like discharge, gleet, coryza with loss of smell and taste, follicular catarrh of the pharynx, thrush with salivation, diphtheria with drowsiness, inflammation of uvula with elongation, catarrh of the bladder, impotence, prostatic fluid, paralysis, chorea, chlorosis, insomnia, pneumonia with loose rattling phlegm, intermittent fever, especially after abuse of quinine. Anasarca, gout, chronic swellings of lymphatic and sebaceous glands. Hemicrania.

Salt or sodium chloride is an essential trace element. This remedy is mainly used for emotional problems where the person has closed down due to suppressed grief or emotional problems.

Natrum mur. types are sensitive, responsible and refined. They tend to dwell on things, harbouring grievances and will cry in private. They dislike fuss and prefer to be independent with bouts of unpredictable behaviour. Persons needing this remedy are serious and inflexible. Easily wounded by criticism, they may become introverted and self-reliant.

Natrum mur patients appear dark or fair skinned, with watery eyes. They can be pear-shaped. Their skin is puffy and greasy and they may be prone to cracks in the centre of the lower lip. Usually these patients are fond of salt.

They are worse between 9.00 a.m. and 11.00 a.m. and in the hot sun.

Natrum mur. is used to treat watery colds, headaches, anaemia, constipation, and backache. Weak areas of the body include the digestive tract, blood, muscles, skin and the mind.

When there is a disturbance or deficiency of the molecules of this salt, which attracts water, the water which should go to the cells remains in the intercellular fluids and hydræmic states ensue, that may be shown in various ways; patients tire easily, are chilly, have cold extremities and often an abnormal craving for salt. Malnutrition, emaciation, secretions of clear, watery fluid, tears, or clear, watery mucus. Clean, frothy tongue. Watery blisters and blebs. Coryza, clear, watery or frothy; watery eyes and much sneezing. Waterbrash, heart-burn. Intermittent fever; Dropsy. Puffiness; Mucous membranes may be abnormally dry.

This remedy has proved curative in intermittent fever, coryza, chlorosis, "whites", leucorrhœa, leukæmia, chlorosis, adynamic states, aphthæ, asthma, bronchitis, catarrhs, coughs, effusions, hay- fever, headache, diarrhœa, watery blisters, constipation, deafness, watery brash, house-maid's knee, hydrocele, neuralgia, pleurisy, rheumatism, sycosis, etc., when the general conditions of Natrum Mur. are in evidence, as noted above.

A deficiency of Natrum Mur makes a person feel very weak and very thirsty. This dryness brings on a throbbing headache that feels like hundreds of little hammers hammering away inside. Coughing during a headache makes one feel like the head were going to burst wide open. The feet feel leaden and it feels like there's a tight band around the lungs. There's a fluttery feeling around the heart with intermittent heartbeats and sometimes, you can feel the pulse all over the body. Very often, one dose brings great relief.

NATRUM PHOSPHORICUM

Synonyms - Nat Phos. Natri Phosphas. Phosphas Natricus. Sodae Phosphas. Sodii Phosphas.

Common Name - Phosphate of Soda.

Chemical Properties - Formula, Na2HPO4, I2H2O. Sp. gravity, 1.55. It is prepared by neutralizing orthophosphoric acid with carbonate of sodium, and is also made from bone-ash. It crystallizes in large, transparent, monoclinic prisms containing twelve molecules of water of crystallization. It has a mild, cooling, saline taste. It is soluble in two parts of hot and in six of cold water. It is insoluble in alcohol. Solutions are slightly alkaline.

Preparation - The pure phosphate of soda is triturated as directed under Class VII, American Pharmacopeia. (Should be kept well corked)

Indications - gastric and intestinal disorders with sour and acid symptoms, worms, acidity, diarrhoea.

Facial Signs:

Greasy, dull shine on the forehead

Greasy nose, T zone

Big skin pores

Blackhead

Pimple

Pale mucous membranes

Hanging cheeks

Double chin

Tongue yellowish in the back

Hanging Cheeks

Where excess skin in the jowl area appears to hang lower than the jawbone.

Greasy or Dull Shine on the Forehead

Greasy or Dull Shine on the Nose

Large Skin Pores

Blackheads and Other Pimples

Pale Mucous Membranes [Nostril Cavities]

Double Chin

Yellowish Coating at the Back of the Tongue

Sodium phosphate is the great pH balancer in the body and is one of the most effective natural antacids there is. Whenever there is more acid than necessary in your body, your digestion suffers and there's heartburn, flatulence, sometimes constipation, sometimes diarrhea. All this adds up to your metabolic rate not being what it should with the result of more weight than what should be your optimum weight as well as water retention – which also adds to your weight. If you are looking for fast weight loss, Nat Phos is not for you – it's a remedy that prides itself on being slow and sure. So no quick weight loss with Nat Phos but it's steady weight loss till you reach your optimum weight – and the great thing is, the weight stays off!

Through the presence of this salt, lactic acid is decomposed in carbonic acid and water. It eliminates the carbonic acid through the lungs. It has also the power to eliminate any excess of sugar from the blood.

This is the remedy in all cases where there is an excess of lactic acid. It acts also upon the bowels, glands, lungs and abdominal organs. Deficiency of this salt in the gastric juice will bring about acid and sour fermentations, and so it cures sour belching and sour rising of fluids. Sour vomiting, sour eructation with flatulence, greenish, sour smelling, diarrhoea, colic, spasms due to acid conditions of the stomach. Fever from acidity of stomach in children. Febrile condition with acid and sour smelling perspiration. Ague with characteristic coating of the tongue. Thick, moist, golden yellow coating of the tongue and palate and also a creamy yellowish exudation are the characteristic symptoms calling for this remedy. Eye complaints discharging a creamy yellow matter. Intestinal worms. Incontinence of urine in children with acidity. Atony of bladder, seminal emissions without dreams, leucorrhoea, with creamy or honey coloured or acid and watery discharge, uterine displacements accompanied by rheumatic pains. Goiter, scrofulosis with acid symptoms. Hives, crusta lactea.

This salt is found in the cells of the blood, muscles nerves, brain and intercellular fluids. A departure from the normal in it is characterized generally by "sourness," an excess of lactic acid; sour eructations, or vomiting, or diarrhœa in infants or adults; acidity; uric acid conditions, rheumatism of the joints, gout. Discharges from the eyes, or sores, are yellow and creamy; tongue yellow; throat and tonsils are covered with yellow, creamy coating. Dyspepsia, sour or acid. Perspiration smells sour.

There could be a tendency to gout – with a lot of pain in the big toe – or rheumatism of the joints, the tongue and the tonsils are covered with a creamy yellow coating which screams 'excess acid', any discharge from the nose, throat or eyes have that same creamy-yellow color and there's a certain 'sourness' in the perspiration, the saliva, the urine. When the pain in the joints grows less, there's pain in the chest and very often it is this pain caused by acidity that makes people feel they are having a heart attack. Acid reflux also benefit a lot from this cell salt.

Eczema is yet another symptom of excess acid in the body and very often, the Nat Phos eczema manifests itself at the ankles with intolerable itching. A deficiency of this salt also results in diabetes which seems to disappear when this salt is given, washing out the excess sugar in the blood as it were.

Through the presence of this salt, lactic acid is decomposed in carbonic acid and water. It eliminates the carbonic acid through the lungs. It has also the power to eliminate any excess of sugar from the blood.

This salt has proved to be curative in indigestion, hyperacidioty, acid stomach, flatulence, sour risings, nausea, vomiting, worms, loss of appetite, diarrhœa, headache, heart-burn, intermittent fever, morning sickness, scabs yellow, sores etc., when the general conditions noted-above are present.

NATRUM SULPHURICUM

Synonyms - Sodium Sulphate. Sodae Sulphas. Sodii Sulphas.

Common Name - Glauber's Salt. Sulphate of Soda.

Chemical Properties - Formula, Na2SO4, 10H2O. It occurs rather abundantly in nature: sea water, saline springs, Russian salt lakes, etc. It is prepared by the action of sulphuric acid on common salt and purified by recrystallization. It forms large, colourless, transparent, oblique, rhombic or six-sided prisms, having a cooling, bitter, saline taste. They effloresce in warm air at 30 °C. They melt in their own water of crystallization, melting also freely at 33 °C; above or below that temperature the solubility decreases.

Preparation - The pure sulphate of sodium is triturated as directed under Class VII, American Pharmacopoeia.

Indications - hepatic diseases, bilious attacks, intermittent fevers, headaches, diarrhoea, diabetes, asthma, la grippe, dropsy.

Facial Signs:

Green-yellow complexion, especially forehead and temples

Bluish redness in the nose

Bluish redness in front of the ears

Redness in the external corner of the eye

Tongue looks dirty and greenish

Redness Only in the Exterior Corners of the Eyes

When only the outside corners or points where the two eyelids [upper and lower] meet, there will be strong and notable redness.

Greenish Yellow Complexion Especially in the Forehead or Temples

Bluish Redness on the Nose

Bluish Redness in Front of the Ears

Tongue Will Have a Dirty or Greenish Appearance

This salt aids and regulates the excretion of the superficial water. It eliminates and excess of water from the blood. It keeps the bile in normal consistency. The three natrum salts work in the body as follows. Natrum Phos creates the water by splitting up of lactic acid; Nat Mur distributes the water through the system. Nat. Sulph. regulates the quantity of water in the organism. Nat. Sulph. is preeminently a liver remedy. It exhibits a marked similarity to the uric acid diathesis and is certainly a valuable remedy in combating or numerous phases of that malady. Dirty, brownish green or grayish- green coating on the root of the tongue. Dark greenish stools from excess of bile, bitter taste, vomiting of bile, diabetes from jaundice, bilious headache, dropsy, diseases of the liver. Excellent in influenza, intermittent fever and ague in all stages with vomiting and other bilious symptoms. Enlargement of the liver, erysipelas, smooth, red shiny eruptions coming in blotches with swelling of skin. Gravel, sand in urine, gout, fig warts, asthma and dyspnoea aggravated by change to damp weather, edematous inflammations of the skin, skin diseases with moist, yellowish scales, yellow watery secretions in all vesicles. Vomiting in pregnancy with bitter taste, fistulous abscesses discharging watery secretions, tendency to warts around the eyes, scalp, face, chest and arms etc. Symptoms are worse in the morning, in damp, wet weather and from lying on left side. Relief in warm dry weather and in the open air.

A person who needs Nat Sulph is usually worse in wet, rainy weather and there's a lot of yellowness in the discharges – the urine, thick, yellow, lumpy discharges from the nose and if it progresses to jaundice, then yellow skin and eyes.

When things get bad, there's always a sick bilious rising from the stomach and the mouth has a bitter taste. Nat Sulph is a great remedy for fever that keeps coming and going, especially for dengue fever and all types of infectious fevers.

The action of this salt is the reverse of that of Natrum Mur., whose action is to attract the needed water to the cells; Natrum Sulph., on the contrary, eliminates waste matter and water. When there is a disturbance in its action, it is shown by a tongue of yellowish green or a dirty brown; discharges the same general colour; biliousness; bitter taste; vomiting, of bitter water or bile; bilious diarrhœa; bilious fever; "yellow fever;" soreness in the region of the liver; jaundice. Worse from wet weather, dampness, moisture, etc. Better in dry and warm surroundings.

This remedy has proved curative in biliousness, bilious colic, jaundice, liver disorders, bilious headache, sick headache, vomiting bile, eructations bitter, diabetes, diarrhœa, dropsy, intermittent fever, yellow fever, dengue, swamps fever, coast fever, vertigo, etc., when the above-mentioned general conditions are shown.

SILICEA

Synonyms - Silica. Silica Tera. Silex. Decarbonized white pebble. Acidium Silicicum. The proper name is Silicic: Oxide.

Common Names - Pure Flint or Quartz. Silicious Earth.

Chemical Properties - Formula, SiO_2. Prepared by fusing silica and carbonate of sodium; dissolving residue filtered and precipitated by hydrochloric acid. It is a white powder, having neither taste nor smell.

Preparation - Pure Silica is triturated according to Class VII, American Pharmacopoeia. Dr P. Wilde uses preferably the silicate of soda known as "liquid glass," which is freely soluble in water.

Indications - chronic suppurations and ulcerations, carbuncles, tonsillitis, glandular swellings, indurations, scrofula, foot sweats, uterine disorders.

Facial Sign:

Shining skin, as varnished (polished shine)

Waxy yellow or pale skin colour

Deep-recumbent eyes

Slip eyelids

Laughter lines

Crow's-feet

Convulsions of the eyelids

Small skin pores

Vertical wrinkles in front of the ears

Brittle hair

Dry nose

Deep Wrinkles

Deep folds or wrinkles such as crow's feet, laugh lines or vertical folds in front of the ears are the main signs of a silica deficiency.

Shining Skin [Entire Face]

Waxy Yellow or Pale Skin

Deep Recumbent Eyes [Indicates a Long-Term Deficiency]

Convulsions of the Upper Eyelids

Convulsions of the Inner Section of Lower Eyelids

Small Skin Pores

Brittle Hair

Dry Nose

It acts more upon the organic substances of the body, involving prominently bones, joints, glands, skin and mucous surfaces, producing malnutrition and corresponding to the scrofulous diathesis. Its action is deep and long lasting. It is especially suited to imperfectly nourished constitutions. It is a remedy for deep-seated chronic and acute suppurations and ulcerations, affecting the tendons, periosteum and bone. promotes suppuration. Indicated when there is hardness and indurations with suppuration. Infiltrations terminating in suppuration. It ripens abscesses by promoting suppurations. Valuable also in diseases resulting from suppressed foot sweats. Metrorrhagia in menstruation, associated with icy coldness over the whole body. Constipation and fetid foot-sweats. Ozena, carbuncles, tonsillitis, scrofula, syphilitic indurations, glandular swellings which become hard and threaten to suppurate. Styes on eyelids. Epilepsy especially nocturnal arid with change of moon. Gouty deposits in large joints of fingers. Chronic dyspepsia, copious night sweats especially in phthisis. Third stage of tuberculosis. Symptoms are always worse at night, during full moon, in the open air and from suppressed foot sweats and are better by the application of heat and warmth.

Silicea is a constituent of the connective tissue, the skin, hair and nails. Disturbances in this element are closely connected with pus formation and fistulous openings; the skin is unhealthy and easily suppurates; the nails are dry and brittle and the hair falls out and is dry; perspiration is offensive, the feet emit a bad smell, and so do the arm-pits; atrophy of parts. Internal chilliness, sensitive to cold air, wants to wrap up warm. In headache must wrap up the head warm.

This element has proved curative in fistula, boils, carbuncles, gouty deposits, rheumatism, hip joint disease, running sores, indurations, perspiration of the feet, pus secretions of a rather watery nature, suppurations, styes, ulcers, whitlows, chilblains, headache, etc., where the above general conditions are present.

You cannot mistake a person whose body needs Silicon Dioxide – he'll stick his feet out of the covers at night even when it's cold because of burning soles. A few doses of Silicon Dioxide are all it takes to feel all right again. This is a great salt that helps the body get rid of any organic matter that is superfluous in the body. Once this is flushed out as waste, the body goes back to feeling normal. The cleansing process could be a bit slow if there are years of accumulated waste and toxins – but Silicon Dioxide goes about it efficiently and thoroughly. It is the body's vacuum cleaner and it throws out all the waste in pus-filled boils or any area that has a septic condition. Silicon Dioxide is great at the beginning of hip-joint disease and using it regularly can reverse the condition in the early stages.

7

Bio-combinations

Combination of Bioplasgens, their ingredients and indications as per Dr. Willmar Schwabe are given below:

No.	Disease	Composition	Condition
1.	Anaemia	Calcarea phos-3x Ferrum phos-3x Natrum mu r-3x Kalium phos-3x In equal proportion	Lack of blood due to indigestible food and to living in unhealthy quarters.Continuous loss of blood from any part of the body. Cerebral and spinal anaemia. A general wasting of the tissues, waxy appearance of the skin; chlorosis, palpitation, tremor and weakness. Anaemia of the brain from prolonged mental strain.Poor digestion, general wasting,neurasthenia, mental and physical depression, and worries

2.	Asthma	Kalium phos-3x Magnesia phos-3x Natrum mur-6x Natrum sulph-3x In equal proportion	Nervous asthma accompanied by cough, gasping, irregular pulse. Asthma with troublesome flatulence or spasms, convulsive tickling cough. Bronchial asthma with yellow sputum, worse in the evening and in warm rooms, better in cool air. Bronchial asthma, dyspnoea(short breath) on going upstairs, dry tickling cough, spasmodic cough, whooping cough.
3	Colic	Magnesia phos-3x Calcarea phos-3x Natrum sulph-3x Ferrum phos-3x Kalium phos-3x In equal proportion	Colics of infants that cause them to draw up their legs, especially during teething. Colic of children and adults from blockage of the intestines caused by flatulence or constipation with formation of gas. Spasmodic pains.

			Flatulent colic, colic due to inflammatory conditions, colic in children during teething or due to flatulence and constipation.
4	Constipation	Calcarea fluor-3x Kalium mur-3x Natrum mur-3x Silicea-3x Calcarea phos-3x In equal proportion	Bowels constipated without apparent cause, liver torpid, stools dry, and black; dull headache; foul breath and bad taste in mouth, tongue coated. Bowels constipated, dry, hard stool, dull headache, foul breath, coated tongue.
5	Coryza	Ferrum phos-3x Kalium mur-3x Natrum mur-6x Kalium sulph-3x In equal proportion	Pain in the head, sneezing, continuous thick white discharge from the nose or discharge from the bronchial tubes due to an irritation and severe inflammation of

			the mucous membranes. Fever, white or grey coated tongue. Inflammatory, febrile catarrhal conditions, coryza with dull headache, sneezing watery discharge.
6	Cough Cold& Catarrh	Ferrum phos-3x Kalium mur-3x Magnesia phos-3x Natrum mur-6x Kalium sulph-3x Natrum sulph-3x In equal proportion	Cold in the head; acute catarrh, rattling hollow cough; painful respiration, pain in chest, bronchitis. Indicated in acute inflammatory, febrile, catarrhal conditions, cough, cold and headache.
7	Diabetes	Magnesia phos-3x Calcarea phos-3x Ferrum phos-3x Kalium phos-3x Natrum phos-3x Natrum sulph-3x In equal proportion	Increased micturition, pain in calves, thirst, dry lips, sleeplessness, nervous prostration. All chronic cases with liver disorders. Recommended as a remedy to support the patient's state of health by

			assimilating the glucose. The kidney and nerve functions impaired by diabetes are improved. It is indicated to relieve many conditions associated with diabetes. It helps better assimilation of glucose.
8	Diarrhoea	Calcarea phos-3x Ferrum phos-3x Kalium phos-3x Kalium sulph-3x Natrum sulph-3x In equal proportion	Thin watery stools with undigested food, thirst, caused by fat or too rich food. White coated tongue. Prostration. Recommended in convalescence. Diarrhoea during dentition, thin water y, greenish stool foul smell with undigested food. Stool with blood or yellow, loose morning stool, which at times is involuntary while passing flatus.

9	Dysentery	Ferrum phos-3x Kalium mur-3x Kalium phos-3x Magnesia phos-3x In equal proportion	Dysentery with mucus and blood. Both painful and painless dysentery.
10	Enlarged tonsils	Calcerea phos-3x Ferrum phos-3x Kalium mur-3x In equal proportion	Inflammed tonsils, follicular tonsillitis, painful with white coating or grayish white patches on tongue or tonsils, bad breath with loss or lowered appetite.
11	Fever	Ferrum phos-3x Kalium mur-3x Kalium sulph-3x Natrum sulph-3x Natrum mur-3x In equal proportion	Inflammatory condition, generally cover all febrile conditions.
12	Headache	Ferrum phos-3x Kalium sulph-3x Magnesia phos-3x Natrum mur-3x Kalium phos-3x	Headaches due to congestion and a rush of blood to the head, neuralgia. Better from heat, worse from cold. Nervousness as a consequence of worries sleeplessness, or a low-functioning liver. Worse in the evening or in a warm room, better in the open air.

13	Leucorrhoea	Kalium mur-6x Ferrum phos-3x Calcarea phos-3x Kalium phos-3x Kalium sulph-3x Natrum mur-3x Calcarea sulph-3x In equal proportion	Discharge like white of egg, acrid and watery. Indicated for general weaknessof young girls with or without functional disturbance.
14	Measles	Ferrum phos-3x Kalium mur-3x Kalium sulph-3x In equal proportion	Sneezing and thin discharge from nose, eyes watery,throbbing headache, cough and fever.
15	Menstrual troubles	Calcarea phos-3x Ferrum phos-3x Kalium phos 3x Magnesia phos-3x Kalium sulph-3x In equal proportion	Irregular menses, bright red if earl y, dark red if late, scanty in young girls, profuse in elderly women.
16	Nervous exhaustion	Calcarea phos-3x Ferrum phos-3x Kalium phos-3x Magnesia phos-3x Natrum mur-3x In equal proportion	Lassitude, depression, nervousness, irritability, loss of impaired memory, confusion, sleeplessness and psychosomatic disorders.

17	Piles	Calcarea fluor-3x Ferrum phos-3x Kalium mur-3x Kalium phos-3x In equal proportion	Bleeding haemorrhoids, fissures, backache, it helps in all kinds of piles.
18	Pyorrhoea	Calcarea fluorica-3x Calcarea sulph-3x Silicea-6x	Gum boil, unnatural looseness of the teeth, with or without pain, toothache, gums sensitive to cold, abscess at root of teeth, spongy bleeding gums, pusin gums and foul.
19	Rheumatism	Ferrum phos-3x Kalium sulph-3x Magnesia phos-3x Natrum sulph-3x Calcarea phos-3x In equal proportion	Articular and muscular rheumatism, inflammatory and febrile complaints, stiff neck, rheumaticpain in shoulder, shifting, wanderingpains, twitching, writer's and player's cramp,cracking of joints, lumbago and sciatica.

20	Skin Diseases	Calcarea fluor-6x Calcarea sulph-3x Kalium sulph-3x Natrum mur-6x Natrum sulph-3x In equal proportion	Acne, cracks, whitlow, eczema, eruptions on the scalp, seborrhea, psoriasis, herpes.
21	Teething Troubles	Calcarea phos-3x Ferrum phos-3x In equal proportion	Tardy dentition and troubles, appetite and digestion are improved, builds the body.
22	Scrofula	Calcarea phos-3x Ferrum phos-3x Kalium mur-3x Silicea-6x In equal proportion	It almost covers all symptoms of both dry and suppurating scruphulous glandular abscesses.
23	Toothache	Calcarea fluor-3x Ferrum phos-3x Magnesia phos-3x Kalium mur- 3x Kalium phos-3x Silicea-6x In equal proportion	Recommended especially in neuralgic cases. Favourable effect in rheumatic toothache. It has a definite role in dental health care covering its malnutrition, toothache, hard swelling of jaw bone, gum boil, unnatural loosing of tooth in their

			sockets and toothache if food or water touches the teeth. Also ulceration of teeth, swelling of glands of face, throat and neck.
24	Tonic for (Five nerve & phos) brain	Calcarea phos-3x Ferrum phos-3x Kalium phos-3x Magnesia phos-3x Natrum phos-3x In equal proportion	The combined Phosphates promote tissue building and provide necessarynutrition of nerves, brain and bones. A general tonic for all chronic wasting diseases, anaemia, general debility and exhaustion with lack of vitality.
25	Acidty Flatulence Indigestion	Magnesia phos-3x Natrum phos-3x Natrum sulph-3x Silicea-6x In equal proportion	Gastric disturbances, hyperacidity. Sour eructation, flatulence, flatulent colic, dyspepsia, bilious vomiting, heart burn and jaundice.

26	Easy Parturition	Calcarea fluor-3x Ferrum phos-3x Calcarea phos-3x Kalium phos-3x Magnesia phos-3x In equal proportion	If taken during the entire time of pregnancy these tablets will greatly relieve the pains of labour. They also favour the mothers general state of health and assist in the development and health of the child. They may also prevent miscarriage.
27	Lack of Vitality	Kalium phos-3x Calcarea phos 3x Natrum mur-6x Natrum phos-3x Ferrum phos-3x Natrum sulph-6x In equal proportion	Symptoms suggestive of impotence, diminished sexual desire, lassitude, general debility, quick emission followed by trembling, weakness and nervousness.
28	General Tonic	Calcerea phos-3x Calcerea fluo r-6x Kalium mur-3x Kalium phos-3x Kalium sulph-3x Ferrum phos-3x Magnesia phos-3x	Helpful in consumption debilitating diseases, for convalescents. It builds up entire system by

	Natrum phos-3x Natrum mur-6x Natrum sulph-3x Silicea-3x Calcarea sulph 3x In equal proportion	providing necessary tissue nutrition. Improved resistance to diseases, helps better utilization of food.

Bibliography

1. CRC Handbook of Chemistry & Physics by Istvan Pais, J. Benton Jones Jr. (18th Ed.).
2. The Elements Third Edition, John Emsley, Clarendon Press, Oxford (1998).
3. Diet and Health, Commission on Life Sciences, National Research Council, National Academy Press, Washington, D.C. (1989).
4. Clinical Nutrition of the Essential Trace Elements and Minerals, John D. Bogden and Leslie M. Klevay. Humana Press, Totowa, New Jersey (2000).
5. The Twelve Tissue Remedies of Schuessler, William Boericke and Willis A. Dewey, Third Edition, Boericke & Tafel, USA (1893).
6. The Zodiac and the Salts of Salvation by George W. Carey, Martino Fine Books (2013).
7. Astrology may be bogus, but the month you're born really seems to matter for your health By Ana Swanson, The Washington Post, June 15, 2015.
8. The Salts of Life: Remedies and Astrological Associations by Karen Bartlett, Lulu Press (2011).
9. Jansky, R.C. How to Use the Cell Salts. Astro-Analytics Publications: Van Nuys, California, (1977).
10. Materia Medica for the New Age Man by Dr. Debasish Kundu, Dr Anton Jayasuriya, Dr. M Ahmed, Originals, New Delhi, (2015).

Notes on Spagyrics

By Dr. Debasish Kundu

Rs. 395/- US $ 21.50 Paperback

In this book author briefly discusses the principles of Alchemy with some exceptional notes on Sexual and Spiritual Alchemy.

CONTENTS: Note to the Readers, Foreword, Preface, Introduction, History of Alchemy, Spagyrics, Principles of Spagyrics, The Quest for the Quintessence, Plant Alchemy, Energetic Spagyrics, The Three Philosophical Principles, Spagyric Electro-Homoeopathy, Energy in the Organism, Herbal Medicine, Spiritual Alchemy, Sexual Alchemy, Spagyric Meditation, Hermetic Philosophy, Fermentation and Distillation of Wine Spirit, Spagyric Experiments, Explanation of Some Spagyrics Terms, Bibliography

Materia Medica and Practice of Medicine in Electro-Homoeopathy

By Dr.Debasish Kundu

Rs. 395/- US $ 21.50 Paperback

CONTENTS: Foreword, Preface, Electrohomoeopathy-An Introduction, Life History of Count Cesare Mattei, Preparation of Electro Homoeopathic Remedies, Electrohomoeopathy Formulas, Constitution and Temperament, Materia Medica of Electrohomoeopathy Medicines, Examination of the Patient, General Rules for Using the Medicines, Practice of Medicine, Points for External Application, Chief Points and their Uses, Clinical Index, Bibliography

Treatise on Spagyric Homoeopathic Pharmacy

By Dr. Debasish Kundu & Dr. Vijay Kant Agnihotri, Sr. Scientist, CSIR, Forewordеd By Prof. Raffaele Pezzani, University of Padova, Italy

Rs. 395/- US $ 21.50 Paperback

It features all necessary information about the method of preparations and formulations of Zimpel, Krauss and Bernus. It is the only book which has incorporated Spagyrics formulas of Zimpel brought back from the lost fragments of time.

According to Prof. Pezzani, it is definitely a valuable guide, a friend that every Electrohomeopathy (according to Mattei) practitioner should possess. It is a must have collection for everyone.

CONTENTS: Dedication, Foreword, Preface, Spagyric Homeopathic Pharmacy, Electrohomoeopathy Formulas, Spagyrics after Zimpel, Krauss and Bernus, Medicinal Plants, Tables of Essential Oil Yielding Plants, Bibliography

Materia Medica for the New Age Man

By Dr. Debasish Kundu, Dr A.Jayasuriya, Chancellor, The Open International University, Colombo and Edited by Dr. M Ahmed, Member, Bangladesh Homeopathy Board, Dhaka

Rs. 450/- US $ 24.50 Hardbound

This is the only book which covered all therapeutic schools of Homeopathy, from Gemmotherapy, Lithotherapy, Bach flower to Spagyric Homeopathy.

CONTENTS: Foreword to the Second Edition, Introduction, Introduction to Homeopathy, Evolution of Disease, Introduction to Vital Force, Miasms, Homeopathic Pharmacy, Case Taking, Doctrine of Dosage, Therapeutic Schools of Homeotherapeutics at a Glance, Nosodes and Sarcodes, Materia Medica, Clinical Index of Homeopathic Remedies, Mother Tinctures (External Use), Do's and Don'ts for Patients, Clinical Tips for Dummies, General Index of Remedies, References

Treatise on Electro-Homoeopathic Pharmacy

By Dr. Debasish Kundu & Dr.Ajit Singh, Foreworded By Prof. Fabio R Ambrosi, Chairman, Mattei Archieves, Italy

Rs. 195/- US $ 15.50 Paperback

CONTENTS: Foreword, Preface, Introduction to Electro Homoeopathic Pharmacy, Laboratory Equipments Used in Electro Homoeopathy Pharmacy, Vehicles used in Electrohomoeopathy, Sources of Electro Homoeopthic Medicines, Collection of Medicinal Plants, Cohobation: An Extraordinary Pharmacy, Methods of Preparation of Spagyric Medicines, Quality Control Procedures, Pharmacodynamics of Electrohomoeopathy Essences, Dosages and Mode of Administration, List of Medicinal Plants Used in

Electrohomoeopathic Remedies, Appendix 1: Terminology, Appendix 2: Prescription Writing, Appendix 3: Biographies, Appendix 4: Apparatus, Bibliography

Essentials of Acupuncture

By Dr. Debasish Kundu & Prof. Choo Led Sin, Chairman, International Federation of Acupuncture, Singapore

Rs. 995/- US $ 40.00 Hardbound

The Only Book which deals with Acupuncture Anaesthesia

CONTENTS: Preface, Introduction, History of Acupuncture, Philosophy of Acupuncture, Five Elements Theory, Diagnosis in Traditional Chinese Medicine, Evaluation and Diagnosis, The Concept of Qi, Management & Research on Some Disorders, How Acupuncture Works, Acupuncture Anesthesia, Laser Acupuncture, Auriculotherapy, Atlas of Acupuncture Points, Therapeutics of Common Ailments, Therapeutics of Common Ailments, Infertility, Impotence and Acupuncture, Acupuncture in Hairfall, Does Acupuncture Hurts, Related Therapies, Explanation of Some Terms, Marmapuncture, Bibliography

Cesare Mattei's Principles of Electro Homeopathy

Interpreted & Revised By Dr. Debasish Kundu

Rs. 395/- US $ 21.50 Paperback

The classic text has been Rewritten in simple language with much needed Interpretation & Revision. In some places the original French edition has been consulted, also enriched with footnotes wherever necessary.

CONTENTS: Preface by Editor, What is Electro-Homeopathy?, Names of the Electro-Homeopathic Remedies, General Information about the Electro-Homeopathic Remedies, Sphere of Action of the Remedies in Globules, General Remarks on the Electric Liquids, Their Mode of Application, Results of Experience, Doses and Method of Administration of the Remedies in Globules, Of Diagnosis, Principles and Rules for the Selection of the Appropriate Remedy, Easy Experiments for Beginners, Catalogue of Diseases Cured by Electro-Homeopathy, Appendix

Stepping Stones to Electo-Homoeopathy (Count Mattei's System of Medicine)

By A J L Gliddon(Original Edition with Vitiation of Blood and Lymph Theory)

Rs. 395/- US $ 21.50 Paperback

A brief insight into the discovery of electro homeopathy together with a rational explanation of the principles involved and the proposed medicines.

CONTENTS: Introduction , The Human Body, Count Mattei's Theories, Symptoms of Disease, The Electro-Homceopathic Remedies, The Globule Remedies, The Electricities, External Use of Electricities, External Use of Globules, Baths, Compresses, etc., How to Select the Remedies, How to Determine the Dose, Dilutions, Dry Globules, Table of Doses, Minute Doses, Effects of the Remedies, Other Hygienic Helps, Diet, Dress, Pure Air, etc.

Essentials of Trace Elements & Biochemic Medicine

By Prof. Dr. Debasish Kundu, Edited By Prof. Seyed Farzin Hassanzadeh Salehian Ph.D. (Iran)

Rs. 350/- US $ 19.00 Paperback

Cell Salts or Bioplasgens have always been considered an important part of healing in Homeopathy and Spagyrics. This book contains all essential materials concerning Trace Elements & Bioplasgen and their relationship with Spagyrics, Clinical Materia Medica with useful suggestions.

CONTENTS: Preface, Introduction to Trace Elements & Bioplasgens, The Functions of The Cell, Astrology and Bioplasgens, Minerals, Trace Elements, Materia Medica of the Bioplasgens, Bio-combinations, Bibliography

A Textbook on Food, Nutrition and Dietetics

By Dr. Debasish Kundu Editor Dr. Malik A.K. Awan Ph.D. (London), Associate Editor Prof. Seyed Farzin Hassanzadeh Salehian Ph.D.(Iran)

Rs. 495/- US $ 20.00 Paperback

CONTENTS: Preface, Relationship between Food, Nutrition & Health, History of Nutrition, Functions of Food, Digestion of Food, Food and Nutrition, Nutrition, Diet & Development, Nutrition & Diet Therapy, Nutrition for Infants, Children, Adults, Women and Elderly, Ideal Diet Plan, The Food Pyramid, Therapeutic Diet, Bibliography

Notes on MJT (Forensic Medicine & Toxicology)

By Dr. Debasish Kundu Ph.D. Assisted By Dr. Ravi Justin Raj NMD, LLB Edited By Dr. Malik A.K. Awan B.S., M.S. (Psychology), D.C.L., D.D. (U.S.A.), Ph.D. (London)

Rs. 550/- US $ 22.00 Paperback

CONTENTS: Part I: Forensic Medicine: Dedication , Preface , Introduction, Scope of Forensic Medicine, Aspects of Identification, Medico-legal Aspects of Death, Investigation of Death, Death by Asphyxia, Medico-legal Aspects of Injuries, Investigation of Wounds, Medico-legal Aspects of Sex Crimes, Medico-legal Aspects of Abortion, Forensic Pathology, Forensic Entomology, Radiation Poisoning, Medico-legal Sections in IPC, Cr PC, AND IE A, Part II: Toxicology: Introduction to Toxicology, General Approach to a Victim of Poison, Clinical Toxicology Laboratory, Practical Aspects of Analytical Toxicology, Toxicants of Public Health Hazard, Medical Toxicants, Environmental Toxicants, Abuse of Drugs, Natural Toxicants, Annexure I: Preparations of Reagents, Annexure II: Apparatuses, Annexure III: Glossary of Terms Used, Annexure IV: Abbreviations Used, Bibliography

Notes on Minor Surgery

By Dr. Debasish Kundu Ph.D. Guided & Edited by Dr. A.K. Banerjee M.B.B.S., M.D. (U.S.A.)

Rs. 395/- US $ 21.50 Paperback

CONTENTS: Part-I: Preface, Acharya Sushruta, Basic Surgical Procedures, Surgery of Some Common Conditions, Part II: Sterilisation, Suture Materials, Nomenclature of Operations, Planning for Operation, Anaesthesia,Operative Surgery, Postoperative Complications, Abscess Drainage, Venesection (Cut Down), Skin Grafting, Circumcision, Vasectomy, Hyderocele, Inguinal Hernia, Strangulated Inguinal Hernia, Femoral Hernia, Umbilical Hernia, Appendicetomy,

Abdominal Incisions, Peptic Ulcer, Vagotomy, Gastrojejumnostomy, Partial Gastrectomy, Closure of Perforated Peptic Ulcer, Right Hemicolectomy, Colostomy, Cholecystectomy, Choledocholithotomy (Supraduodenal), Spleenectomy, Lumbar Sympathectomy, Haemorrhoidectomy, Suprapubic Cystostomy, Prostatectomy, Exposure of Kidney , Exposure of the Ureter and Ureterolithotomy, Mastectomy, Thyroidectomy, Tracheostomy, Empyema Thoracis, Amputations, Bibliography

Principles and Practice of Naturopathy

By Dr. Debasish Kundu Editor Dr. Malik A. K. Awan Ph.D. (London) Associate Editor Prof. Sayed Farzin Hassanzadeh Salehian Ph.D.(Iran)

Rs. 750/- US $ 30.00 Paperback

CONTENTS: Foreword, Preface to the First Edition, Preface to the Third Edition, Naturopathy: Its Principles & Pioneers, Physiology, Food and Nutrition, Hygiene and Sanitation, Biology, Herbology, Medicinal Plants, Magnet Therapy, Yoga and Meditation, Massage Therapy, Medical Gymnastics, Chemistry, Bacteriology, Toxicology, Pathology, Osteology, Neurology, Ethics, Hydro Therapy and Helio Therapy, Colour Therapy, Fasting and Diet, Mud Therapy and Fango Therapy, Acupressure, Aromatherapy, Reflexology, Iridology, Vitamins and Balanced Diets, Bibliography

Diseases of Women (Adopted from Margaret Seifert's Krankheiten Der Franen)

By Dr. Shefalika Kundu, Edited By Dr. Debasish Kundu & Dr. Sudeshna Kundu

Rs. 350/- US $ 19.00 Paperback

The book is intended as a handbook on diseases of women with their Electrohomeopathic treatment. Besides an update on the literature on Contraception using Spagyrics , entirely new topics Anatomy of Uterus and Stages of development in Pregnancy are added.

CONTENTS: Preface to the Second Edition, Foreword to the First Edition, Preface, Introduction, Anatomy and Physiology of Sexual Organs of Women, General View of Treatment, Diseases and Their Treatment, Hygienic Care of the Body and Toilet, Anatomy of Uterus in Pregnancy, Notes on Various Diseases, Family Planning, Contraception in Electrohomoeopathy,Diet, Index of Diseases Discussed, Bibliography

Lectures on Materia Medica & Therapeutics

By Dr. H. D. Banerjee, Foreworded By M V Mattei, Thoroughly Revised & Edited By Prof. Dr. Debasish Kundu

Rs. 225/- US $ 18.00 Paperback

CONTENTS: Preface to the Third Edition, Preface to the Second Edition, Foreword to the First Edition, Introduction, On Electro-Homoeopathic Principles, On Principles of Orthodox School, On Homeopathic Principles , On Objections to Electro-Homoeopathy, Chemical Analysis of the Remedies, Dynamisation of the Remedies, On Minute Doses, On Frequency of the Doses, Purgatives in Electro-Homoeopathy, On Prescription Writing, Materia Medica & Therapeutics, On Therapeutics of the Remedies

Principles & Art of Cure in Electrohomeopathy

By Prof. Dr.Debasish Kundu Ph.D.

Rs. 195/- US $ 15.00 Paperback

CONTENTS: Introduction to Electrohomeopathy, Philosophy, The Discoverer, Principles of Nature, Introduction to Electrohomeopathy Medicines, The Iris science, Sources and preparation of Electrohomeopathy Medicines, Cohobation, Spagyric Tinctures, Classification of Electrohomeopathy Medicines, Classification, Preparation and Therapeutics uses of Electrohomeopathy Medicines, Potentisation of Electrohomeopathy Medicines and Electric fluids, Preparation and Therapeutic uses of Ointments and Lotions, Points for application Electric Fluids, Ointments and Lotions, Plain talks on using the medicines, Potentisation and Bio-Magnetism, The Similia of Electrohomeopathy, The Scientific basis of Electrohomeopathy System of Medicine, World's present day need of Electrohomeopathy, Clinical Index.

A Clinical Treatise on Cancer

By Prof. Dr.Debasish Kundu Ph.D. Forewored By Dr. B.B. Upreti, Ph. D. General Secretary, All Nepal Electro-Homeo Medical Association, Hetauda, Nepal

Rs. 195/- US $ 15.00 Paperback

CONTENTS: Introduction, The Increase of Cancer and it's Causes, The Treatment of Cancer, Diet for Patients, Hygienic Care of the Patients

Books Published By LBO Publishing, 700 N Valley St., Suite B PMB 11884 Anaheim, CA 92801, USA Marketed In India Exclusively By Originals, Delhi

Pharmacodynamics in Spagyric Medicine(Plant Alchemy)

By Dr. Debasish Kundu & Dr.Sudeshna Kundu, Edited by Gisela Bruckel(Germany), El Akrem Hayouni (Tunisia), Forwarded by Dr.Peter Morrell (U.K.), Prof. Luigi Vernacchia & Dr.Fabio Ambrosi (Italy)

Printed on Art Paper, USD ($) 70.00, Hardbound

It is the only trusted book to learn Sacred Alchemical Philosophy with Practical Laboratory Spagyrics, it covers from history & principles of Alchemy to the rarest topic Botanical Consciousness in Spagyrics, besides, Alchemy and the Zodiac Connection and how Spagyric Medicines work. In addition, detailed Pharmaceutical Process which are being carried out in most modern laboratories : from Apparatus, Vehicles, Sources of Medicines, Preparation of Spagyric Essences, quality control like Phytochemical Analysis, etc. , all major Spagyric Methods known to mankind, incl., Mattei, Zimpel, Junius, Solaris, Krauss,etc., besides the sacred Indian, Arabian and Chinese methods, Doctrine of Dosage, and much more. An Encyclopedia of Spagyrics or Plant Alchemy in one nutshell.

This work is edited by Gisela Bruckel, who is a Pharmacist and her Pharmacy in Wurzburg was the Main Dealer of Mattei Remedies in Europe till M V Mattei era, and Prof. El Akrem Hayouni, World famous authority on Plant Alchemy.

CONTENTS: Foreword, Preface, Part 1: Introduction to Spagyric Medicine, History of Alchemy, Principles of Spagyrics, The Simila of Alchemy, Difference Between Homoeopathy and Spagyric Homoeopathy, Botanical Consciousness in Spagyrics, Micronutrients and Spagyrics, Alchemy and the Zodiac Connection, How Spagyric Medicines Work, Alchemy and Spagyrics, Spagyrics : The Future in Medicine, Part 2: Pharmacy in Plant Alchemy, Pharmaceutical Process, Laboratory Apparatus, Vehicles Used in Plant Alchemy, Sources of Medicines, Preparation of Spagyric Essence, Spagyric Essence by Cohobation Method, Phytochemical Analysis of Plants, Different Spagyric Methods, Quality Control Procedures, Safety Measures in Laboratory, Doctrine of Dosage, Medicinal Plants, Terminology, Appendix, Bibliography

Mysticism, Romance & Secrets of Count Cesare Mattei (With Properly Transcripted Secret Formulas)

By Prof. Dr. Debasish Kundu , Ph.D. (U.S.A.)

Printed on Art Paper, USD ($) 40.00 Hard Bound

It is the Bible of Mattei Electrohomoeopathy : covering the true life of Cesare Mattei and properly transcripted Empirical Formulas & Secret Pharmacy of Electrohomoeopathy, incl. Medicinal Plants Used by Cesare Mattei.

Contributors-Prof. Raffaele Pezzani, University of Padova, Italy, Dr. Fabio R. Ambrosi, University of Sapienza, Rome, Italy, Prof. El Akrem Hayouni, University of Manouba, Tunisia, Allesandro Rapparini, Vice Pres., Archivio Museo Cesare Mattei, Bologna, Italy, Prof. Peter Morrell, Formerly Honorary Research Associate, History of Medicine, Staffordshire University, U.K., Dr. Terry Mitchell, Alchemist & Director, Phylak GmbH, U.K., Willow Morningsky, Spagyrist & Psychologist, Southern Oregon University, Ashland, Oregon, U.S.A. etc.

CONTENTS: Introduction, Dedication, Note to the Readers, Acknowledgements, Alchemist's Prayer, Preface, The Castle of Love, The Mystery Unveiled, Emerald Tablet of Cesare Mattei, Mysticism & Romance of Cesare Mattei, Electro Homoeopathy Pharmacology, Medicinal Plants Used by Cesare Mattei, Glossary of Pharmacological Terms, Bibliography

For Further Information and Ordering:
Originals/Low Price Publications
A-6, Second Floor, Nimri Commercial Centre,
Ashok Vihar Phase-4, Delhi - 110 052 (India)
Tel.: +91 11 2730 2453 Fax: 011 4706 1936
Mobile: 98100-12366
Website: www.Lppindia.com,
e-mail: info@Lppindia.com
info@Lbopub.com